D1357368

Fluoride in Drinking-water

World Health Organization titles with IWA Publishing

Water Quality: Guidelines, Standards and Health edited by Lorna Fewtrell and Jamie Bartram. (2001)

WHO Drinking-water Quality Series

Assessing Microbial Safety of Drinking-water: Improving Approaches And Methods edited by Al Dufour, Mario Snozzi, Wolfgang Koster, Jamie Bartram, Elettra Ronchi and Lorna Fewtrell. (2003)

Fluoride in Drinking-water edited by K. Bailey, J. Chilton, E. Dahi, M. Lennon, P. Jackson and J. Fawell. (2006)

Protecting Groundwater for Health: Managing the Quality of Drinking-water Sources edited by Oliver Schmoll, Guy Howard, John Chilton and Ingrid Chorus. (2006)

Safe Piped Water: Managing Microbial Water Quality in Piped Distribution Systems by Richard Ainsworth. (2004)

Water Treatment and Pathogen Control: Process Efficiency in Achieving Safe Drinking-water by Mark W LeChevallier and Kwok-Keung Au. (2004)

WHO Emerging Issues in Water and Infectious Disease Series

Heterotrophic Plate Counts and Drinking-water Safety: The Significance of HPCs for Water Quality and Human Health edited by J. Bartram, J. Cotruvo, M. Exner, C. Fricker, A. Glasmacher. (2003)

Pathogenic Mycobacteria in Water: A Guide to Public Health Consequences, Monitoring and Management edited by S. Pedley, J. Bartram, G. Rees, A. Dufour and J. Cotruvo. (2004)

Waterborne Zoonoses: Identification, Causes and Control edited by J.A. Cotruvo, A. Dufour, G. Rees, J. Bartram, R. Carr, D.O. Cliver, G.F. Craun, R. Fayer, and V.P.J. Gannon. (2004)

Water Recreation and Disease: An Expert Review of the Plausibility of Associated Infections, their Acute Effects, Sequelae and Mortality edited by K. Pond. (2005)

For further details contact: **Portland Customer Services**, Commerce Way, Colchester, Essex, CO2 8HP, UK.
Tel: +44 (0) 1206 796351; Fax: +44 (0) 1206 799331; Email: sales@portland-services.com;
or order online at: **www.iwapublishing.com**
Also available from WHO Press, World Health Organization, 20 Avenue Appia, 1211 Geneva 27, Switzerland
(tel.: +41 22 791 3264; fax: +41 22 791 4857; e-mail: bookorders@who.int); http://www.who.int/bookorders

Fluoride in Drinking-water

J. Fawell, K. Bailey, J. Chilton, E. Dahi,
L. Fewtrell and Y. Magara

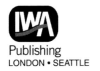

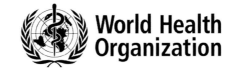

Published on behalf of the World Health Organization by
IWA Publishing, Alliance House, 12 Caxton Street, London SW1H 0QS, UK

Telephone: +44 (0) 20 7654 5500; Fax: +44 (0) 20 7654 5555; Email: publications@iwap.co.uk
www.iwapublishing.com

First published 2006
© World Health Organization (WHO) 2006
Printed by TJ International (Ltd), Padstow, Cornwall, UK

British Library Cataloguing-in-Publication Data
A CIP catalogue record for this book is available from the British Library

WHO Library Cataloguing-in-Publication Data
Fluoride in drinking-water / J. Fawell ... [et al.].

      1.Fluorides. 2.Fluorides - adverse effects. 3.Potable water - standards. 4.Environmental exposure. 5.Water - analysis. 6.Water purification. 7.Guidelines. I.Fawell, J. II.World Health Organization.
ISBN 92 4 156319 2   (NLM classification: QV 282)
ISBN 978 92 4 156319 2

ISBN13: 9781900222969 (IWA Publishing)
ISBN 1900222965 (IWA Publishing)

Table of contents

Acknowledgements

Special thanks are due to the following whose work was crucial in the development of this monograph on Fluoride in Drinking-water either as authors or in providing detailed comments on specific sections.

Dr K. Bailey, WRc-NSF Ltd, Medmenham, UK (since retired).

Dr J. Bartram, Water, Sanitation and Health, WHO, Geneva, Switzerland.

Dr D. Chapman, Department of Zoology, Ecology and Plant Science, University College Cork, Ireland for extensive contribution to the editing process.

Dr Bingheng Chen, School of Public Health, Fudan University Shanghai, China.

Dr J. Chilton, British Geological Survey, Wallingford, UK.

Dr J. Cotruvo, J. Cotruvo Associates, Washington, D.C., USA.

Prof. Eli Dahi, EnDeCo, Environmental Development Cooperation Group, Soborg, Denmark for extensive contributions including the new information on costs in Chapter 5.

Mr J. Fawell, Independent Consultant, High Wycombe, UK, acted as coordinator.

Dr L. Fewtrell, Centre for Research into Environment & Health, (CREH), University of Wales, University College, Lampeter, UK.

Dr J. Fitzgerald, Department of Human Services, Adelaide, Australia.

Dr G. Howard, Department for International Development (DFID) Bangladesh, Dhaka, Bangladesh (formerly of Water Engineering and Development Centre, Loughborough University, UK).

Dr P. Jackson, WRc-NSF Ltd, Medmenham, UK.

Dr G. Karthikeyan, Department of Chemistry, The Gandhigram Rural Institute, Tamilnadu, India.

Prof. M. Lennon, School of Dentistry, University of Liverpool, UK.

Dr R. Kfir, Chief Executive Officer, Water Research Commission, South Africa.

Ms V. Ngowi, Tropical Pesticides Research Institute, Tanzania.

Dr J. Schoeman, Council for Scientific and Industrial Research (CSIR), South Africa.

Dr Quangyong Xiang, School of Public Health, Fudan University, Shanghai, China.

Many others also provided comments without which it would not have been possible to complete this document.

1

Introduction

The first WHO publication dealing specifically with drinking-water quality was published in 1958 as *International Standards for Drinking-water* (WHO, 1958). It was subsequently revised in 1963 and in 1971 under the same title (WHO, 1963, 1971). In 1984–85, the first edition of the WHO *Guidelines for Drinking-water Quality* was published. The philosophy and content of the Guidelines constituted a significant departure from the previous International Standards. The basic premise of the Guidelines was that they are not standards as such, but should be used as a basis for setting national or regional standards taking into account local social, cultural, environmental and economic considerations.

In 1989, work was started on a second edition of the *Guidelines for Drinking-water Quality* (GDWQ) which was published in three volumes: *Volume 1 Recommendations* (WHO, 1993), *Volume 2 Health Criteria and Other Supporting Information* (WHO, 1996) and *Volume 3 Surveillance and Control of Community Supplies* (WHO, 1997) with Addenda published in 1998 and 2002 (WHO, 1998, 2002). A fully revised edition of *Volume 1 Recommendations* was published in 2004 (WHO, 2004).

The primary aim of the *Guidelines for Drinking-water Quality* is the protection of public health. The GDWQ provide an assessment of the health risk presented by micro-organisms and chemicals present in drinking-water. This assessment can then be applied to the development and implementation of national standards for drinking-water quality. In addition, in response to demands from Member States, the Guidelines have always included guidance material concerning specific problems related to small community supplies.

Fluoride is one of the very few chemicals that has been shown to cause significant effects in people through drinking-water. Fluoride has beneficial effects on teeth at low concentrations in drinking-water, but excessive exposure to fluoride in drinking-water, or in combination with exposure to fluoride from other sources, can give rise to a number of adverse effects. These range from mild dental fluorosis to crippling skeletal fluorosis as the level and period of exposure increases. Crippling skeletal fluorosis is a significant cause of morbidity in a number of regions of the world. Fluoride is known to occur at elevated concentrations in a number of parts of the world and in such circumstances can have, and often has, a significant adverse impact on public health and well-being. There is now a continuing process of updating the GDWQ, through which it was concluded that there was a need for a monograph on fluoride in drinking-water that would be useful to a wide range of individuals, including health workers and sanitary engineers who may require a broad introduction to the subject, but would still provide more detailed guidance in some specific areas. Such a monograph could provide an appropriate introduction and background information, and indicate where other more detailed information could be obtained. The primary focus of the monograph should be the prevention of adverse effects from excessive levels of fluoride in drinking-water. This document, *Fluoride in Drinking-water*, was written to meet that need. It is one of several monographs, which also cover arsenic and complements guidance previously published on cyanobacteria in water. The draft monograph was issued for extensive consultation and the final draft, which considered the comments received, also received further peer review from experts in developing and developed countries.

1.1   References

WHO 1958 *International Standards for Drinking-Water*. World Health Organization, Geneva.
WHO 1963 *International Standards for Drinking-Water*. World Health Organization, Geneva.
WHO 1971 *International Standards for Drinking-Water*. World Health Organization, Geneva.
WHO 1993 *Guidelines for Drinking-water Quality. Volume 1. Recommendations.* 2nd edition World Health Organization, Geneva.
WHO 1996 *Guidelines for Drinking-water Quality. Volume 2. Health Criteria and Other Supporting Information.* 2nd edition. World Health Organization, Geneva.
WHO 1997 *Guidelines for Drinking-water Quality. Volume 3. Surveillance and Control of Community Supplies.* 2nd edition. World Health Organization, Geneva.
WHO 1998 *Guidelines for Drinking-water Quality. Volume 3. Addendum. Surveillance and Control of Community Supplies.* 2nd edition. World Health Organization, Geneva.

WHO 2002 *Guidelines for Drinking-water Quality. Volume 3. Addendum. Surveillance and Control of Community Supplies*. 2nd edition. World Health Organization, Geneva.
WHO 2004 *Guidelines for Drinking-water Quality. Volume 1. Recommendations*. 3rd edition. World Health Organization, Geneva.

2

Environmental occurrence, geochemistry and exposure

Fluorine is the lightest member of the halogen group and is one of the most reactive of all chemical elements. It is not, therefore, found as fluorine in the environment. It is the most electronegative of all the elements (Hem, 1989) which means that it has a strong tendency to acquire a negative charge, and in solution forms F^- ions. Other oxidation states are not found in natural systems, although uncharged complexes may be. Fluoride ions have the same charge and nearly the same radius as hydroxide ions and may replace each other in mineral structures (Hem, 1985). Fluoride thus forms mineral complexes with a number of cations and some fairly common mineral species of low solubility contain fluoride.

Fluorine in the environment is therefore found as fluorides which together represent about 0.06–0.09 per cent of the earth's crust. The average crustal abundance is 300 mg kg^{-1} (Tebutt, 1983). Fluorides are found at significant levels in a wide variety of minerals, including fluorspar, rock phosphate, cryolite, apatite, mica, hornblende and others (Murray, 1986). Fluorite (CaF_2) is a common fluoride mineral of low solubility occurring in both igneous and sedimentary rocks. Fluoride is commonly associated with volcanic activity and fumarolic gases. Thermal waters, especially those of high pH, are also rich in fluoride (Edmunds and Smedley, 1996). Minerals of commercial importance include cryolite and rock phosphates. The fluoride salt cryolite is used for the production of aluminium (Murray, 1986) and as a pesticide (USEPA, 1996). Rock phosphates are converted into phosphate fertilizers by the removal of up to 4.2 per cent fluoride (Murray, 1986); the removed and purified fluoride (as fluorosilicates) is a source of fluoride that in some countries is added to drinking-water in order to protect against dental caries (Reeves, 1986, 1994).

2.1   Fluoride distribution in water

Fluoride is found in all natural waters at some concentration. Seawater typically contains about 1 mg l^{-1} while rivers and lakes generally exhibit concentrations of less than 0.5 mg l^{-1}. In groundwaters, however, low or high concentrations of fluoride can occur, depending on the nature of the rocks and the occurrence of fluoride-bearing minerals. Concentrations in water are limited by fluorite solubility, so that in the presence of 40 mg l^{-1} calcium it should be limited to 3.1 mg l^{-1} (Hem, 1989). It is the absence of calcium in solution which allows higher concentrations to be stable (Edmunds and Smedley, 1996). High fluoride concentrations may therefore be expected in groundwaters from calcium-poor aquifers and in areas where fluoride-bearing minerals are common. Fluoride concentrations may also increase in groundwaters in which cation exchange of sodium for calcium occurs (Edmunds and Smedley, 1996).

Fluorosis has been described as an endemic disease of tropical climates, but this is not entirely the case. Waters with high fluoride concentrations occur in large and extensive geographical belts associated with a) sediments of marine origin in mountainous areas, b) volcanic rocks and c) granitic and gneissic rocks. A typical example of the first extends from Iraq and Iran through Syria and Turkey to the Mediterranean region, and hence from Algeria to Morocco. Other important examples come from the southern parts of the USA, southern Europe and the southern parts of the former USSR.

The most well-known and documented area associated with volcanic activity follows the East African Rift system from the Jordan valley down through Sudan, Ethiopia, Uganda, Kenya and the United Republic of Tanzania. Many of the lakes of the Rift Valley system, especially the soda lakes, have extremely high fluoride concentrations; 1,640 mg l^{-1} and 2,800 mg l^{-1} respectively, in the Kenyan Lakes Elmentaita and Nakuru (Nair et al., 1984), and up to 690 mg l^{-1} in the Tanzanian Momella soda lakes. In Kenya, a detailed survey of fluoride in groundwater was undertaken by Nair et al. (1984). Of over 1,000 groundwater samples taken nationally, 61 per cent exceeded 1 mg l^{-1}, almost 20 per cent exceeded 5 mg l^{-1} and 12 per cent exceeded 8 mg l^{-1}. The volcanic areas of the Nairobi, Rift Valley and Central Provinces had the highest concentrations, with maximum groundwater fluoride concentrations reaching 30–50 mg l^{-1}. Most of the sampled wells and boreholes were providing drinking-water, and the prevalence of dental fluorosis in the most affected areas was observed to be very high (Manji and Kapila, 1986). A similar picture emerges for the United Republic of Tanzania, where 30 per cent of waters used for drinking exceeded 1.5 mg l^{-1} fluoride (Latham and Gretch, 1967) with concentrations in the Rift Valley of up to 45 mg l^{-1}.

High groundwater fluoride concentrations associated with igneous and meta-morphic rocks such as granites and gneisses have been reported from India, Pakistan, West Africa, Thailand, China, Sri Lanka, and Southern Africa. In China, endemic fluorosis has been reported in all 28 provinces, autonomous regions and municipalities except Shanghai. Both shallow and deeper groundwaters are affected; in general the deeper groundwaters have the higher concentrations. In Sri Lanka, Dissanayake (1991) found concentrations of up to 10 mg l^{-1} in groundwaters in the Dry Zone, associated with dental and possibly skeletal fluorosis. In the Wet Zone, the intensive rainfall and long-term leaching of fluoride and other minerals from the crystalline bedrock are probably respon-sible for the much lower concentrations. Reported drinking-water fluoride levels are outlined on a country-by-country basis in Chapter 7.

Endemic fluorosis remains a challenging and extensively studied national health problem in India. In 1991, 13 of India's 32 states and territories were reported to have naturally high concentrations of fluoride in water (Mangla, 1991), but this had risen to 17 by 1999 (UNICEF, 1999). The most seriously affected areas are Andhra Pradesh, Punjab, Haryana, Rajasthan, Gujarat, Tamil Nadu and Uttar Pradesh (Kumaran, *et al.*, 1971; Teotia *et al.*, 1984). The highest concentration observed to date in India is 48 mg l^{-1} in Rewari District of Haryana (UNICEF, 1999). The high concentrations in groundwater are a result of dissolu-tion of fluorite, apatite and topaz from the local bedrock, and Handa (1975) noted the general negative correlation between fluoride and calcium concentrations in Indian groundwater.

Efforts to address the problem of fluoride in rural water supplies in India have been led by the Rajiv Ghandi National Drinking Water Mission, with consider-able support from external agencies, particularly UNICEF. However, even with the great interest in fluoride in India, it is not easy to arrive at an accurate or reli-able estimate of the number of people at risk. This is because of the difficulty of sampling groundwater from India's many millions of handpumps. Existing sampling has been selective but unstructured, taking some villages from districts and some of the many pumps in each village (UNICEF, 1999). Further, there have been no comprehensive health surveys for dental fluorosis from which the overall extent of the problem could be assessed. Nevertheless, in the most affected states listed above, half or more of the districts have some villages with groundwater supplies having high fluoride concentrations. In these states, 10 to 25 per cent of the rural population has been estimated to be at risk, and perhaps a total of 60–70 million people in India as a whole may be considered to be so (UNICEF, 1999).

2.2   Exposure

2.2.1 Air

Due to dust, industrial production of phosphate fertilizers, coal ash from the burning of coal and volcanic activity, fluorides are widely distributed in the atmosphere. However, air is typically responsible for only a small fraction of total fluoride exposure (USNRC, 1993). In non-industrial areas, the fluoride concentration in air is typically quite low (0.05–1.90 μg m^{-3} fluoride) (Murray, 1986). In areas where fluoride-containing coal is burned or phosphate fertilizers are produced and used, the fluoride concentration in air is elevated leading to increased exposure by the inhalation route. High levels of atmospheric fluoride occur in areas of Morocco and China (Haikel *et al.*, 1986, 1989). In some provinces of China, fluoride concentrations in indoor air ranged from 16 to 46 μg m^{-3} owing to the indoor combustion of high-fluoride coal for cooking and for drying and curing food (WHO, 1996). Indeed, more than 10 million people in China are reported to suffer from fluorosis, related in part to the burning of high fluoride coal (Gu *et al.*, 1990).

2.2.2 Dental products

A number of products administered to, or used by, children to reduce dental decay contain fluoride. This includes toothpaste (1.0–1.5 g kg^{-1} fluoride), fluoride solutions and gels for topical treatment (0.25–24.0 g kg^{-1} fluoride) and fluoride tablets (0.25, 0.50 or 1.00 mg fluoride per tablet), among others. These products contribute to total fluoride exposure, albeit to different degrees. It is estimated that the swallowing of toothpaste by some children may contribute about 0.50 or 0.75 mg fluoride per child per day (Murray, 1986).

2.2.3 Food and beverages other than water

Vegetables and fruits normally have low levels of fluoride (e.g. 0.1–0.4 mg kg^{-1}) and thus typically contribute little to exposure. However, higher levels of fluoride have been found in barley and rice (e.g. about 2 mg kg^{-1}) and taro, yams and cassava been found to contain relatively high fluoride levels (Murray, 1986).

In general, the levels of fluoride in meat (0.2–1.0 mg kg^{-1}) and fish (2–5 mg kg^{-1}) are relatively low. However, fluoride accumulates in bone and the bones of canned fish, such as salmon and sardines, which are also eaten. Fish protein concentrates may contain up to 370 mg kg^{-1} fluoride. However, even

Table 2.1   Levels of fluoride in foodstuffs

Food	Fluoride conc. (mg kg^{-1})[a]	Comment	References
Milk and milk products	0.01–0.8	Range of concentrations in 12 varieties of dairy products in Canada	Dabeka and McKenzie (1995)
	0.045–0.51	Range of mean concentrations in 13 varieties of dairy products in Hungary	Schamschula et al. (1988a)
	0.019–0.16	Range of concentrations in milk and milk products sampled between 1981 and 1989 in Germany	Bergmann (1995)
Meat and poultry	0.04–1.2	Range of concentrations in 17 varieties of (cooked and raw) meat and poultry in Canada	Dabeka and McKenzie (1995)
	0.01–1.7	Range of mean concentrations in 7 varieties of meat and poultry in Hungary	Schamschula et al. (1988a)
	0.29	Mean concentration in canned meat and sausage sampled between 1981 and 1989 in Germany	Bergmann (1995)
Fish	0.21–4.57	Range of concentrations in 4 varieties of fish available in Canada	Dabeka and McKenzie (1995)
	0.06–1.7	Range of concentrations in 6 varieties of fish available in the USA	Whitford (1996)
Soups	0.41–0.84	Range of concentrations in 4 varieties of soup available in Canada	Dabeka and McKenzie (1995)

Continued

Table 2.1 Continued

Food	Fluoride conc. (mg kg^{-1})[a]	Comment	References
Soups cont.	0.42–0.94	Range of mean concentrations in 7 varieties of soup available in Hungary	Schamschula et al. (1988a)
Baked goods and cereals	0.04–1.02	Range of concentrations in 24 varieties of baked goods and cereals available in Canada	Dabeka and McKenzie (1995)
	1.27–1.85	Range of mean concentrations in rice consumed in three villages in China	Chen et al. (1996)
	0.06–0.49	Range of mean concentrations in 13 varieties of baked goods and cereals available in Hungary	Schamschula et al. (1988a)
	0.05–0.39	Range of concentrations in bread and grains sampled between 1981 and 1989 in Germany	Bergmann (1995)
Vegetables	0.01–0.68	Range of concentrations in 38 varieties of raw, cooked and canned vegetables in Canada	Dabeka and McKenzie (1995)
	0.28–1.34	Range of mean concentrations in three staple vegetables consumed in three villages in China	Chen et al. (1996)
	0.01–0.86	Range of mean concentrations in 24 varieties of vegetables available in Hungary	Schamschula et al. (1988a)
	0.023	Mean concentration in some vegetables sampled between 1981 and 1989 in Germany	Bergmann (1995)

Continued

Table 2.1 Continued

Food	Fluoride conc. (mg kg^{-1})[a]	Comment	References
Fruits and fruit juices	0.01–0.58	Range of concentrations in 25 varieties of fruit and fruit juices available in Canada	Dabeka and McKenzie (1995)
	0.03–0.19	Range of mean concentrations in 16 varieties of fruits and fruit juices available in Hungary	Schamschula et al. (1988a)
	0.02–2.8	Range of concentrations in 532 varieties of fruit juice and juice-flavoured beverages in the USA	Kiritsy et al. (1996)
	0.027	Mean concentration in some fruits sampled between 1981 and 1989 in Germany	Bergmann (1995)
	0.014–0.35	Range of concentrations in some fruit juices sampled between 1984 and 1989 in Germany	Bergmann (1995)
Fats and oils	0.05–0.13	Range of concentrations in 3 varieties of fats and oils available in Canada	Dabeka and McKenzie (1995)
Sugars and candies	0.01–0.28	Range of concentrations in 7 varieties of sugar-containing products available in Canada	Dabeka and McKenzie (1995)
	0.01–0.31	Range of mean concentrations in 12 varieties of sugar-containing foods available in Hungary	Schamschula et al. (1988a)
Beverages	0.21–0.96	Range of concentrations in 6 varieties of beer, wines, coffee and soft drinks available in Canada	Dabeka and McKenzie (1995)

Continued

Table 2.1   Continued

Food	Fluoride conc. (mg kg^{-1})[a]	Comment	References
Beverages cont.	0.19–0.78	Range of mean concentrations in 3 varieties of coffee and soft drinks available in Hungary	Schamschula et al. (1988a)
	0.003–0.39	Range of concentrations in some soft drinks sampled between 1984 and 1989 in Germany	Bergmann (1995)
	0.02–1.28	Range of concentrations in 332 samples of soft drinks sold in Iowa, USA, between 1995 and 1997	Heilman et al. (1999)
Tea	4.97	Concentration in tea available in Canada	Dabeka and McKenzie (1995)
	90.94–287.9	Range of mean concentrations of tea consumed in three villages in China	Chen et al. (1996)
	243.7	Mean concentration in 4 samples of tea leaves used in Hungary	Schamschula et al. (1988a)
	82–371	Range of concentrations in samples of 32 tea leaves purchased in Hong Kong	Wei et al. (1989)
	0.005–0.174	Range of concentrations in herbal and children's teas sampled between 1984 and 1989 in Germany	Bergmann (1995)
	0.37–2.07	Range of concentrations in black tea sampled between 1984 and 1989 in Germany	Bergmann (1995)

[a] For liquid items, concentrations are in mg l^{-1}

Source: IPCS (2002)

Table 2.2   Concentrations of fluoride in infant foods[a]

Food item	Fluoride concentration (µg l^{-1})[b]	References
Human milk	5–10	Esala et al. (1982); Spak et al. (1983); Ekstrand et al. (1984)
Cow's milk	30–60	J. Ekstrand (unpublished data)
Formula		
Ready to feed	100–300	Johnson and Bawden (1987); McKnight-Hanes et al. (1988)
Concentrated liquid		
Milk-based	100–300	
Isolated soybean-based	100–400	
Powdered		
Milk-based	400–1,000	
Isolated soybean-based	1,000–1,600	
Most products other than dry cereals	100–300	Singer and Ophaug (1979); Dabeka et al. (1982)
Fruit juices		
Produced with non-fluoridated water	10–200	Singer and Ophaug (1979); Dabeka et al. (1982)
Produced with fluoridated water	100–1,700	

Continued

Table 2.2 Continued

Food item	Fluoride concentration ($\mu g\ l^{-1}$)[b]	References
Dry cereals		
Produced with non-fluoridated water	90–200	Singer and Ophaug (1979); Dabeka et al. (1982)
Produced with fluoridated water	4,000–6,000	
Wet-pack cereal fruit products	2,000–3,000	Singer and Ophaug (1979); Dabeka et al. (1982)
Poultry-containing products	100–5,000	Singer and Ophaug (1979); Dabeka et al. (1982)

[a] From Fomon and Ekstrand (1993); Fomon et al. (2000).
[b] Concentration ranges have been rounded off. Most reported values fall within the ranges listed in the table.
Source: IPCS (2002)

Table 2.3   Estimated intakes of fluoride

Sources of fluoride exposure	Age group	Estimated fluoride intake, mg/day (mg kg⁻¹ bw/day)[a]	Comment	References
Foodstuffs	Adults	0.6	Intakes based upon levels of fluoride and consumption of major foodstuffs	Varo and Koivistoinen (1980)
Foodstuffs and drinking-water in four regions of the USA	Infants (6 months): (drinking-water <0.3 mg l⁻¹ fluoride) (drinking-water >0.7 mg l⁻¹ fluoride) Children (2 years old): (drinking-water <0.3 mg mg l⁻¹ fluoride) (drinking-water >0.7 mg l⁻¹ fluoride)	0.226 (0.028) 0.418 (0.052) 0.207 (0.017) 0.621 (0.05)	Intakes based on fluoride levels in market basket survey of foods and drinking-water and estimated consumption	Ophaug et al. (1985)
Foodstuffs (including infant formulas) and beverages, fluoridated or non-fluoridated drinking-water in North America	Children (up to 6 years of age)	0.05–1.23 (0.01–0.16)	Summary of eight studies published between 1943 and 1988 on the estimated intakes of fluoride from food and beverages by North American children	Levy (1994)

Table 2.3 Continued

Sources of fluoride exposure	Age group	Estimated fluoride intake, mg/day (mg kg^{-1} bw/day)[a]	Comment	References
Ambient air, foodstuffs (inc. infant formula or breast-fed), fluoridated or non-fluoridated drinking-water, soil, dentifrice in Canada	Infants (up to 6 months of age)	<0.01–0.65 (<0.001–0.09)	Estimated total intakes by multimedia exposure analysis based upon ranges of mean concentrations of fluoride in ambient air, fluoridated or non-fluoridated drinking-water and soil; levels of fluoride in survey of 109 foodstuffs in Canada, breast milk, infant formula and average level of fluoride in dentifrice available in Canada, as well as assigned reference values for body weight, inhalation of air, and consumption of water, soil and foodstuffs, by various age groups of the population of Canada	Government of Canada (1993)
	Children (7 months to 4 years)	0.6–2.1 (0.05–0.16)		
	Adolescents (5–11 years)	0.7–2.1 (0.03–0.08)		
	Adults (20+ years)	2.2–4.1 (0.03–0.06)		

Table 2.3 Continued

Sources of fluoride exposure	Age group	Estimated fluoride intake, mg/day (mg kg^{-1} bw/day)[a]	Comment	References
(Infant formula or breast-fed), cereal, juices, fluoridated or non-fluoridated drinking-water, dentifrice, fluoride supplements in the USA	Infants (6 months of age)	0.4–1.4 (0.05–0.19)	Estimated intakes based upon concentrations of fluoride in breast milk or various infant formulas reconstituted with fluoridated or non-fluoridated drinking-water, levels in juices and cereals, as well as estimated intakes from dentifrice and fluoride supplements by children in the USA	Levy et al. (1995)
	Children (1 year of age)	0.32–0.73 (0.03–0.08)		
	Children (2–3 years of age)	0.76–1.23 (0.06–0.09)		
Various infant formulas reconstituted with fluoridated or non-fluoridated drinking-water in Australia	infants (6 months of age)	0.13–1.35 (0.02–0.17)	Estimated intakes based upon levels of fluoride in various infant formulas available in Australia reconstituted with either fluoridated or non-fluoridated drinking-water	Silva and Reynolds (1996)
	Infants (1 year of age)	0.14–1.65 (0.02–0.17)		
Ambient air, drinking-water and limited variety of foodstuffs in China	Adolescents (7–15 years)	1.16–4.57	Estimated intakes based upon levels of fluoride in ambient air, local supplies of drinking-water and levels in a limited variety of locally grown foodstuffs in an area	Liu (1995)
	Adults (16+ years)	1.61–7.51		

Continued

Table 2.3 Continued

Sources of fluoride exposure	Age group	Estimated fluoride intake, mg/day ($mg\ kg^{-1}$ bw/day)[a]	Comment	References
			of China with known elevated levels of fluoride in local water supplies	
Ambient air, drinking-water and limited variety of foodstuffs in China	Adolescents (8–15 years)	1.51–10.6	Estimated intakes based upon levels of fluoride in ambient air, indoor air, local supplies of drinking-water and levels of fluoride in a limited variety of locally grown foodstuffs in four areas of China where fluoride-containing coal is burned for heating and cooking	Liu (1995)
	Adults (16+ years)	1.79–17.0		
Principal foods consumed by Tibetan and Han peoples residing in Sichuan province in China (levels of fluoride in drinking-water were low [0.1 mg l^{-1}])	Tibetan (8–15 years) (>15 years)	5.49 10.43	Increased intake of fluoride by Tibetans based upon their consumption of a local type of prepared barley and brick tea; foodstuffs not consumed by Han residing in this area; prevalence of dental and skeletal fluorosis greater among Tibetans than among Han	Cao et al. (1996)
	Han (8–15 years) (>15 years)	1.44 2.54		

Continued

Table 2.3 Continued

Sources of fluoride exposure	Age group	Estimated fluoride intake, mg/day (mg kg^{-1} bw/day)[a]	Comment	References
Ambient air, beverages, food and drinking-water in Hungary	Children with a mean age of 3.9 years	0.22–1.11	Estimated intakes based upon levels in available foodstuffs, beverages, air and drinking-water containing levels of fluoride ranging from 0.06 to 3.1 mg l^{-1}	Schamschula et al. (1988b)
	Adolescents with a mean age of 14 years	0.3–1.49		
Drinking-water and food in India	Children (age not specified)	1.5–20	Estimated range of mean intakes based upon levels in foodstuffs and local supplies of drinking-water that ranged in concentration from 0.32 to 9.6 mg l^{-1}	Karthikeyan et al. (1996)
Drinking-water and food in normal or fluorotic villages in India	Adults (age not specified)	0.84–4.69 (normal) 3.40–27.1 (fluorotic)	Range of intakes based upon consumed foodstuffs and local supplies of drinking-water from rural areas in India considered either normal or fluorotic, based upon the absence or occurrence of endemic skeletal fluorosis in these areas, respectively	Anasuya et al. (1996)

Continued

Table 2.3   Continued

Sources of fluoride exposure	Age group	Estimated fluoride intake, mg/day (mg kg^{-1} bw/day)[a]	Comment	References
Diet, beverages and toothpaste in New Zealand	Children (3–4 years of age)	0.17–1.31 (0.01–0.07)	Range of intakes based on duplicate-diet survey of foodstuffs and beverages (non-fluoridated or fluoridated) consumed as well as calculated intake from toothpaste, in a study of 66 children	Guha-Chowdhury et al. (1996)
Commercially available foods and drinking-water in Germany	Infants 1–12 months of age	0.099–0.205	Estimated intake based upon consumption of commercially available food and drinking-water containing 0.13 mg l^{-1} fluoride	Bergmann (1995); Bergmann and Bergmann (1995)
Breast milk and homemade food in Germany	Infants 1–12 months of age	0.002–0.075 (0.0005–0.007)	Estimated intakes by infants receiving breast milk as well as homemade foods	
Food, beverages and drinking-water in Germany	Children 1–15 years of age	0.112–0.264	Estimated intake based upon consumed foodstuffs, beverages and drinking-water	Bergmann (1995); Bergmann and Bergmann (1995)

Continued

Table 2.3 Continued

Sources of fluoride exposure	Age group	Estimated fluoride intake, mg/day (mg kg^{-1} bw/day)[a]	Comment	References
Foods, beverages and drinking-water in Germany	Adolescents (15–18 years of age)	0.523 (males) (0.008)	Estimated intake based upon consumed foodstuffs, beverages and drinking-water	
		0.470 (females) (0.009)		
Foods, beverages and drinking-water in Germany	Adults	0.560 (males) (0.007)	Estimated intake based upon consumed foodstuffs, beverages and drinking-water	
		0.442 (females) (0.007)		
	16- to 40-month-old children consuming drinking-water containing 0.3 mg l^{-1} fluoride	0.965 (0.073)	Estimated intake based upon consumed foodstuffs, beverages and drinking-water	
Foods, beverages and dentifrice in the USA	16- to 40-month-old children consuming drinking-water containing 0.8–1.2 mg l^{-1} fluoride	0.965 (0.07)	Estimated intake based upon consumed foods, beverages and dentifrice	Rojas-Sanchez et al. (1999)

[a] Data in parentheses are the estimated intakes of fluoride, expressed as mg/kg body weight per day, when presented in the reference cited.

Source: IPCS (2002)

with a relatively high fish consumption in a mixed diet, the fluoride intake from fish alone would seldom exceed 0.2 mg F⁻ per day (Murray, 1986).

Milk typically contains low levels of fluoride, e.g. 0.02 mg l⁻¹ in human breast milk and 0.02–0.05 mg l⁻¹ in cow's milk (Murray, 1986). Thus milk is usually responsible for only a small fraction of total fluoride exposure.

Tea leaves contain high levels of fluoride (up to 400 mg kg⁻¹ dry weight). Fluoride exposure due to the ingestion of tea has been reported to range from 0.04 mg to 2.7 mg per person per day (Murray, 1986). However, some Tibetans have been observed to ingest large amounts of fluoride (e.g. 14 mg per day) due to the consumption of brick tea as a beverage (Cao *et al.*, 1997). This type of tea is made from older leaves and contains much higher levels of fluoride than standard teas such as black or green tea.

It is also possible that other forms of tea will contribute to fluoride uptake, although data appear to relatively limited. In one study 34 per cent of the fluoride in black tea was shown to remain in the oral cavity but no data were presented on absorption from the gastrointestinal tract (Simpson *et al.*, 2001). The fluoride content of a range of different foods is given in Tables 2.1 and 2.2.

In general, Western-style diets appear to contribute only slightly to the total daily fluoride intake (Murray, 1986). However, not everyone eats such a diet. The following examples are exceptional to the general rule:

- Trona ($Na_3H(CO_3)_2.2H_2O$) is used in cooking in the United Republic of Tanzania to tenderize certain vegetables. Fluoride contaminated trona has significantly contributed to the prevalence and severity of dental fluorosis in the United Republic of Tanzania (Mabelya, 1997).
- Consumption of high fluoride brick tea as a beverage (Cao *et al.*, 1997).
- In some regions in China significant dietary fluoride exposure occurs due to the consumption of maize polluted by fly ash generated by the burning of high fluoride coal (Chen, 1991).
- The composition of the diet influences retention of dietary fluoride (Whitford, 1997). High protein diets (e.g. Western-style diet) result in a more acidic urine than a vegetarian diet. A more acidic urine results in increased retention of fluoride due to decreased renal excretion. However, at present, the effects of a vegetarian vs. a non-vegetarian diet on the effects produced by fluoride in different regions of the world are unclear.

2.2.4 *Water*

Drinking-water is typically the largest single contributor to daily fluoride intake (Murray, 1986). However, as noted above, this is not necessarily true in every case (e.g. Haikel *et al.*, 1986, 1989; Chen, 1991; Cao *et al.*, 1997; Mabelya, 1997). For a given individual, fluoride exposure (mg kg⁻¹ of body weight per

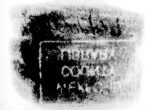

Table 2.4   Daily fluoride intake in different endemic areas of China using
high-fluoride coal for cooking and drying foodstuffs indoors

Endemic area	Coal type	Daily intake (mg/person)			
		Food	Drinking-water	Air	Total
Sichuan	Soft coal	8.86	0.1	0.67	9.63
Hubei	Anthracite	4.12	0.45	0.55	6.12
Jiangxi	Anthracite	2.54	0.5	0.24	3.28
Hunan	Anthracite	1.81	0.52	0.31	2.64
Huber	Anthracite	1.86	0.42	0.15	2.43
Jiangxi (Control)	Firewood	1.14	0.24	0.11	1.49

Source: IPCS (2002)

day) via drinking-water is determined by the fluoride level in the water and the daily water consumption (litres per day). Water consumption data are most readily available for countries such as Canada (Environment Health Directorate, 1977), the USA (Ershow and Cantor, 1989) and the UK (Hopkin and Ellis, 1980). More recently national figures can be obtained or computed from various compendia of environmental and water supply statistics such as World Bank (1994) and WRI (1996). However, national consumption figures, especially for developing countries, may be of limited use for this purpose because there are likely to be major differences between urban communities with fully piped supplies and rural communities using wells and boreholes with handpumps. Consequently, data concerning exposure to fluoride are difficult to come by except for temperate regions. In the USA, young children who consume water containing 0.7–1.2 mg l^{-1} fluoride are estimated to be exposed to approximately 0.5 mg fluoride per day (USNRC, 1993); for those drinking 1 litre of water per day exposure may be up to 1.2 mg fluoride per day (USEPA, 1994). Similar values would probably apply to other similar climatic regions.

For a given individual, water consumption increases with temperature, humidity, exercise and state of health, and is modified by other factors including diet. Roughly, the closer to the Equator, the higher the water consumption (Murray, 1986).

2.2.5 *Total fluoride exposure*

Based on the previous discussion, it follows that total daily fluoride exposure can vary markedly from one region to another. However, from several studies, a rough estimate of total daily fluoride exposure in a temperate climate would be approximately 0.6 mg per adult per day in an area in which no fluoride is added to the drinking-water and 2 mg per adult per day in a fluoridated area (WHO, 1984). In many countries this can be potentially increased for children from the use of fluoridated dental products but there will be significant variation in individual exposure. In hot climates the much higher consumption of water will also increase the intake and this is frequently highly significant. In addition, fluoride exposure in many areas is considerably higher as a consequence of a range of practices, including the consumption of brick tea and the cooking and drying of food with high fluoride coal. A range of estimated fluoride intakes as a consequence of exposure to a number of different sources is given in Tables 2.3 and 2.4.

2.3   References

Anasuya, A., Bapurao, S., and Paranjape, P.K. 1996 Fluoride and silicon intake in normal and endemic fluorotic areas. *Journal of Trace Elements in Medicine and Biology.*, **10**, 149–155.

Bergmann, K.E. and Bergmann, R.L. 1995 Salt fluoridation and general health. *Adv. Dent. Res.*, **9**, 138–142.

Bergmann, R. 1995 *Fluorid in der Ernährung des Menschen*. Biologische Bedeutung für den wachsenden Organismus. Habilitationsschrift. Virchow-Klinikum der Humboldt-Universität, Berlin, 133 pp.

Cao, J., Bai, X., Zhao, Y., Zhou, D., Fang, S., Jia, M., and Wu, J. 1996 The relationship of fluorosis and brick tea drinking in Chinese Tibetans. *Environmental Health Perspectives.*, **104**, 1340–1343.

Cao, J., Bai, X., Zhao, Y., Zhou, D., Fang,S., Jia, M. and Wu, J. 1997 Brick tea consumption as the cause of dental fluorosis among children from Mongol, Kazak and Yugu populations in China. *Food and Chemical Toxicology*, **35**(8), 827–833.

Chen, M.J. 1991 An investigation of endemic fluorine poisoning caused by food contaminated by smoke containing fluorine [Article in Chinese; reference based on English Abstract]. *Chung Hua Yu Fang I Hsueh Tsa Chih*, **25**(3), 171–173.

Chen, Y.X., Lin, M.Q., He, Z.L., Chen, C., Min, D., Liu, Y.Q. and Yu, M.H. 1996 Relationship between total fluoride intake and dental fluorosis in areas polluted by airborne fluoride. *Fluoride*, **29**, 7–12.

Dabeka, R.W. and McKenzie, A.D. 1995 Survey of lead, cadmium, fluoride, nickel and cobalt in food composites and estimation of dietary intakes of these elements by Canadians in 1986–1988. *J. Assoc. Off. Anal. Chem. Int.*, **78**, 897–909.

Dabeka, R.W., McKenzie, A.D., Conacher, H.B.S., and Kirkpatrick, B.S. 1982 Determination of fluoride in Canadian infant foods and calculation of fluoride intake by infants. *Canadian Journal of Public Health*, **73**, 188–191.

Dissanayake, C. B. 1991 The fluoride problem in the groundwater of Sri Lanka - environmental management and health. *International Journal of Environmental Health Studies*, **38**, 137–156.

Edmunds, W.M. and Smedley, P.L. 1996 Groundwater geochemistry and health: an overview. In: Appleton, Fuge and McCall [Eds] *Environmental Geochemistry and Health. Geological Society Special Publication*, **113**, 91–105.

Ekstrand, J., Hardell, L.I. and Spak, C.J. 1984 Fluoride balance studies on infants in a 1-ppm water fluoride area. *Caries Research*, **18**, 87–92.

Environmental Health Directorate 1977 *Tap Water Consumption in Canada*: Ministry of Health and Welfare, 77-EHD-18.

Ershow, A.G. and Cantor, K.P. 1989 *Total Water and Tapwater Intake in the United States: Population-Based Estimates of Quantities and Sources*, National Cancer Institute Order #263-MD-810264.

Esala, S., Vuori, E., and Helle, A. 1982 Effect of maternal fluorine intake on breast milk fluorine content. *British Journal of Nutrition,* **48**, 201–204.

Fomon, S.J. and Ekstrand, J. 1993 Fluoride. In: Fomon, S.J. [Ed.] *Nutrition of Normal Infants*. Mosby, St Louis, Missouri, 299–310.

Fomon, S.J., Ekstrand, J., and Ziegler, E.E. 2000 Fluoride intake and prevalence of dental fluorosis: Trends in fluoride intake with special attention to infants. *Journal of Public Health Dentistry*, **60**, 131–139.

Government of Canada 1993 *Canadian Environmental Protection Act. Priority Substances List assessment report for inorganic fluorides*. Prepared by Health Canada and Environment Canada. Ottawa, Ontario, Canada Communication Group (ISBN 0-662-21070-9).

Gu, S.L., Rongli, J. and Shouren, C. 1990 The physical and chemical characteristics of particles in indoor air where high fluoride coal burning takes place. *Biomedical and Environmental Sciences*, **3**(4), 384–390.

Guha-Chowdhury, N., Drummond, B.K. and Smillie, A.C. 1996 Total fluoride intake in children aged 3 to 4 years — a longitudinal study. *Journal of Dental Research*, **75**, 1451–1457.

Haikel, Y. *et al.* 1986 Fluoride content of water, dust, soils and cereals in the endemic dental fluorosis area of Khouribga (Morocco). *Archives of Oral Biology*, **31**(5), 279–286.

Haikel, Y. *et al.* 1989 The effects of airborne fluorides on oral conditions in Morocco. *Journal of Dental Research*, **68**(8),1238–1241.

Handa, B.K. 1975 Geochemistry and genesis of fluoride-containing groundwaters in India. *Groundwater*, **13**, 275–281.

Heilman, J.R., Kiritsy, M.C., Levy, S.M., and Wefel, J.S. 1999 Assessing fluoride levels of carbonated soft drinks. *J. Am. Dent. Assoc.*, **130**, 1593–1599.

Hem, J.D. 1989 *Study and Interpretation of the Chemical Characteristics of Natural Water*. Water Supply Paper 2254, 3rd edition, US Geological Survey, Washington, D.C., 263 pp.

Hopkin, S.M. and Ellis, J.C. 1980 *Drinking Water Consumption in Great Britain*, Technical Report TR 137, Water Research Centre, Medmenham, UK.

IPCS 2002 *Fluorides*. Environmental Health Criteria 227, International Programme on Chemical Safety, World Health Organization, Geneva.

Johnson, J. Jr and Bawden, J.W. 1987 The fluoride content of infant formulas available in 1985. *Pediatr. Dent.*, **9**, 33–37.

Karthikeyan, G., Pius, S., and Apparao, B.V. 1996 Contribution of fluoride in water and food to the prevalence of fluorosis in areas of Tamil Nadu in south India. *Fluoride*, **29**, 151–155.

Kiritsy, M.C., Levy, S.M., Warren, J.J., Guha-Chowdhury, M., Heilman, J.R., and Marshall, T. 1996 Assessing fluoride concentrations of juices and juice-flavoured drinks. *J. Am. Dental Assoc.*, **127**, 895–902.

Kumaran, P., Bhargava, G. N. and Bhakuni, T.S. 1971 Fluorides in groundwater and endemic fluorosis in Raajasthan. *Indian Journal of Environmental Health*, **13**, 316–324.

Latham, M. C. and Gretch, P. 1967 The effects of excessive fluoride intake. *American Journal of Public Health*, **57**, 651–660.

Levy, S.M. 1994 Review of fluoride exposures and ingestion. *Community Dentistry and Oral Epidemiology,* **22**, 173–180.

Levy, S.M., Kiritsy, M.C., and Warren, J.J. 1995 Sources of fluoride intake in children. *Journal of Public Health Dentistry,* **55**, 39–52.

Liu, Y. [Ed.] 1995 Human exposure assessment of fluoride. An international study within the WHO/UNEP Human Exposure Assessment Location (HEAL) Programme. Beijing, Chinese Academy of Preventive Medicine, Institute of Environmental Health Monitoring, Technical Cooperation Centre of Fluoride/HEAL Programme, 64 pp.

Mabelya, L. 1997 Dental fluorosis and the use of a high fluoride-containing trona tenderizer (magadi), *Community Dentistry and Oral Epidemiology,* **25**(2),170–176.

Mangla, B. 1991 India's dentists squeeze fluoride warnings off tubes. *New Scientist*, **131**, 16.

Manji, F. and Kapila, S. 1986 Fluorides and fluorosis in Kenya. Part 1, The occurrence of fluorides. *Odontostomatol. Trop.*, **9**, 15–20.

McKnight-Hanes, M., Leverett, D., Adair, S., and Shields, C. 1988 Fluoride content of infant formulas: soy-based formulas as a potential factor in dental fluorosis. *Pediatric Dentistry*, **10**, 189–194.

Murray J.J. [Ed.] 1986 *Appropriate Use of Fluorides for Human Health*, World Health Organization, Geneva.

Nair, K.R, Manji, F. and Gitonga, J.N. 1984 The occurrence and distribution of fluoride in groundwaters of Kenya. In: *Challenges in African Hydrology and Water Resources*, Proceedings of the Harare Symposium, IAHS Publ. 144, 75–86.

Ophaug, R.H., Singer, L., and Harland, B.F. 1985 Dietary fluoride intake of 6-month and 2-year-old children in four dietary regions of the United States. *American Journal of Clinical Nutrition,* **42**, 701–707.

Reeves, T.G. 1986 *Water Fluoridation. A Manual for Engineers and Technicians*. United States Department of Health and Human Services, Centres for Disease Control and Prevention, 138 pp.

Reeves, T.G. 1994 *Water Fluoridation. A Manual for Water Plant Operators*. United States Department of Health and Human Services, Centres for Disease Control and Prevention, 99 pp.

Rojas-Sanchez, F., Kelly, S.A., Drake, K.M., Eckert, G.J., Stookey, G.K. and Dunipace, A.J. 1999 Fluoride intake from foods, beverages and dentifrice by young children in communities with negligibly and optimally fluoridated water: a pilot study. *Community Dentistry and Oral Epidemiology,* **27**, 288–297.

Schamschula, R., Duppenthaler, J., Sugar, E., Toth, K. and Barmes, D. 1988a Fluoride intake and utilization by Hungarian children: associations and interrelationships. *Acta Physiologica Hungarica,* **72**, 253–261.

Schamschula, R., Un, P., Sugar, E., and Duppenthaler, J. 1988b The fluoride content of selected foods in relation to the fluoride concentration of water. *Acta Physiologica Hungarica*, **72**, 217–227.

Silva, M. and Reynolds, E.C. 1996 Fluoride content of infant formulae in Australia. *Australian Dental Journal*, **41**, 37–42.

Simpson, A., Shaw, L. and Smith, A.J. 2001 The bio-availability of fluoride from black tea. *Journal of Dentistry*, **29**(1), 15–21.

Singer, L. and Ophaug, R. 1979 Total fluoride intake of infants. *Pediatrics*, **63**, 460–466.

Spak, C.J., Hardell, L.I. and de Chateau, P. 1983 Fluoride in human milk. *Acta Paediatrica Scandinavica,* **72**, 699–701.

Tebutt, T.H. Y. 1983 *Relationship Between Natural Water Quality and Health.* United Nations Educational, Scientific and Cultural Organization, Paris.

Teotia, S.P.S., Teotia, M., Singh, D.P., Rathour, R.S., Singh, C.V., Tomar, N.P.S., Nath, M. and Singh, N.P. 1984 Endemic Fluorosis: change to deeper bore wells as a practical community-acceptable approach to its eradication. *Fluoride*, **17**, 48–52.

UNICEF 1999 *State of the art report on the extent of fluoride in drinking water and the resulting endemicity in India.* Report by Fluorosis Research & Rural Development Foundation for UNICEF, New Delhi.

USEPA 1996 *R.E.D. FACTS, Cryolite*, EPA-738-F-96-016, United States Environmental Protection Agency.

USNRC 1993 *Health Effects of Ingested Fluoride.* National Research Council, National Academy Press, Washington D.C.

Varo, P. and Koivistoinen, P. 1980 Mineral composition of Finnish foods. XII. General discussion and nutritional evaluation. *Acta Agriculturae Scandinavica,* **22**(suppl), 165–171.

Wei, S.H.Y., Hattab, F.N., and Mellberg, J.R. 1989 Concentration of fluoride and other selected elements in teas. *Nutrition*, **5**, 237–240.

Whitford, G. 1996 *The Metabolism and Toxicity of Fluoride,* 2nd edition. Karger, Basel, 156 pp (Monographs in Oral Science, Volume 16).

Whitford, G.M. 1997 Determinants and mechanisms of enamel fluorosis. *Ciba Foundation Symposium*, **205**, 226–241.

WHO 1984 *Fluorine and Fluorides*, Environmental Health Criteria 36. World Health Organization, Geneva.

World Bank 1994 *From Scarcity to Security: Averting a Water Crisis in the Middle East and North Africa.* The World Bank, Washington D.C

WRI (World Resources Institute) 1996 *World Resources, a Guide to the Global Environment: the Urban Environment.* WRI/UNEP/UNDP/WB, Oxford University Press.

3

Human health effects

Fluoride has beneficial effects on teeth at low concentrations in drinking-water, but excessive exposure to fluoride in drinking-water, or in combination with exposure to fluoride from other sources, can give rise to a number of adverse effects. These range from mild dental fluorosis to crippling skeletal fluorosis as the level and period of exposure increases. Crippling skeletal fluorosis is a significant cause of morbidity in a number of regions of the world.

Both national and international groups (USNRC, 1993; IPCS, 2002) have comprehensively reviewed available data on the metabolism and health effects of fluoride in both laboratory animals and humans. The following is a summary of the conclusions that have been developed by these groups, particularly the IPCS working group on fluorides held in May 2001 (IPCS, 2002). The reader is directed to these documents for a more detailed assessment of the data.

3.1 Fluoride metabolism

3.1.1 Absorption

Approximately 75–90 per cent of ingested fluoride is absorbed. In an acidic stomach, fluoride is converted into hydrogen fluoride (HF) and up to about 40 per cent of the ingested fluoride is absorbed from the stomach as HF. High stomach pH decreases gastric absorption by decreasing the concentration uptake

© 2006 World Health Organization (WHO). *Fluoride in Drinking-water* by J. Fawell, K. Bailey, J. Chilton, E. Dahi, L. Fewtrell and Y. Magara. ISBN: 1900222965. Published by IWA Publishing, London, UK.

of HF. Fluoride not absorbed in the stomach is absorbed in the intestine and is unaffected by pH at this site (Whitford, 1997; IPCS, 2002).

Relative to the amount of fluoride ingested, high concentrations of cations that form insoluble complexes with fluoride (e.g. calcium, magnesium and aluminium) can markedly decrease gastrointestinal fluoride absorption (Whitford, 1997; IPCS, 2002).

3.1.2 Distribution

Once absorbed into the blood, fluoride readily distributes throughout the body, with approximately 99 per cent of the body burden of fluoride retained in calcium rich areas such as bone and teeth (dentine and enamel) where it is incorporated into the crystal lattice. In infants about 80 to 90 per cent of the absorbed fluoride is retained but in adults this level falls to about 60 per cent. Fluoride crosses the placenta and is found in mothers milk at low levels essentially equal to those in blood (WHO, 1996; IPCS, 2002).

Under certain conditions, plasma fluoride levels provide an indication of the level of fluoride in the drinking-water consumed. USNRC (1993) notes that *"Provided that water is the major source of fluoride intake, fasting plasma fluoride concentrations of healthy young or middle-aged adults expressed in micromoles per litre are roughly equal to the fluoride concentrations in drinking water expressed as milligrams per litre"*. Levels of fluoride that are found in the bone vary with the part of the bone examined and with the age and sex of the individual. Bone fluoride is considered to be a reflection of long-term exposure to fluoride (IPCS, 2002).

3.1.3 Excretion

Fluoride is excreted primarily via urine (IPCS, 2002). Urinary fluoride clearance increases with urine pH due to a decrease in the concentration of HF. Numerous factors (e.g. diet and drugs) can affect urine pH and thus affect fluoride clearance and retention (USNRC, 1993).

3.2   Effects on laboratory animals and *in vitro* systems

3.2.1 Medium and long-term exposure

A number of sub-chronic and chronic studies have been carried out in laboratory animals in which relatively high doses of soluble fluoride were given in drinking-water. In some studies there is uncertainty regarding the actual dose because commercial laboratory animal rations contain variable amounts of fluoride. Dental fluorosis and a range of effects on bone were noted in several studies. A number of other adverse effects have also been reported, including increased hepatic cell size, nephrosis, myocardial mineralization and degeneration of the seminipherous tubules in testis in mice (IPCS, 2002).

3.2.2 *Mutagenicity and related end-points*

A large number of mutagenicity studies have been conducted with inorganic fluoride ion. This includes studies in bacteria, insects, laboratory animals and *in vitro* studies with human cells. The results have been mixed but, in general, fluoride is not mutagenic in prokaryotes. There have been a number of positive results in a variety of mammalian cell types for chromosome damage (USNRC, 1993; WHO, 1996; IPCS, 2002). It is generally considered that these effects are due to interference with protein synthesis rather than any direct interaction between fluoride and DNA. Although some cytogenetic damage or changes in sperm cell morphology have been reported in rodents following intraperitoneal injection of fluoride, most studies by the oral route are negative (IPCS, 2002). In commenting on these studies, particularly those in human cells, WHO (1996) has concluded that the data are probably of limited relevance for humans.

3.2.3 *Carcinogenicity*

In 1987, the International Agency for Research on Cancer (IARC) reviewed the available data concerning the carcinogenicity of fluoride and concluded that there was inadequate evidence of carcinogenicity in experimental animals (IARC, 1987).

Two separate sets of long-term fluoride carcinogenicity studies in rats and mice have been published in the 1990s (NTP, 1990; Bucher *et al.*, 1991; Maurer *et al.*, 1990, 1993). These studies have been extensively reviewed with the general conclusion that they do not provide adequate evidence to conclude that fluoride is carcinogenic (USNRC, 1993; WHO, 1996; IPCS, 2002).

3.2.4 *Developmental and reproductive toxicity*

Effects on the morphology of reproductive organs and reproductive function have been reported in male and female rabbits and mice given doses of greater than 4.5 mg kg^{-1} body weight per day for varying periods, either orally or by injection. However, in recent studies in laboratory animals, no effects have been observed on reproduction, reproductive organs or the development of the foetus (IPCS, 2002).

3.3   Effects on humans

A number of studies have reported on the acute effects of fluoride exposure following fluoridation overdosing. However, the effects of long-term exposure to naturally occurring fluoride from drinking-water and other environmental sources is the major concern with regard to human health. A large number of epidemiological studies have been conducted in many countries concerning the effects of long-term exposure to fluoride. Information from countries where dental or skeletal fluorosis has been documented is summarized in Chapter 7.

3.3.1 *Effects on teeth*

The beneficial and the detrimental effects of fluoride naturally present in water were well established by the early 1940s. High levels of fluoride present in concentrations up to 10 mg l^{-1} were associated with dental fluorosis (yellowish or brownish striations or mottling of the enamel) while low levels of fluoride, less than 0.1 mg l^{-1}, were associated with high levels of dental decay (Edmunds and Smedley, 1996), although poor nutritional status is also an important contributory factor.

Concentrations in drinking-water of about 1 mg l^{-1} are associated with a lower incidence of dental caries, particularly in children, whereas excess intake of fluoride can result in dental fluorosis. In severe cases this can result in erosion of enamel. The margin between the beneficial effects of fluoride and the occur-rence of dental fluorosis is small and public health programmes seek to retain a suitable balance between the two (IPCS, 2002). The various indices used to rate the severity of dental fluorosis are outlined in the Appendix.

The level of dental caries (measured as the mean number of **D**ecayed, **M**issing or **F**illed teeth) falls from seven at a fluoride concentration of 0.1 mg l^{-1} to around 3.5 at a fluoride concentration of 1.0 mg l^{-1}. As fluoride concentration increased further (up to 2.6 mg l^{-1}) dental decay continues to fall, but only slightly (Dean, 1942; USPHS, 1991). Conversely, dental fluorosis increases as fluoride concentration increases. At a fluoride concentration of 1 mg l^{-1} about 20 per cent of children have evidence of dental fluorosis but this fluorosis is of a mild degree of severity and would not be cosmetically obvious to the children or their parents (Dean, 1942). Thus the evidence suggested that, at least for fluoride naturally present in water, the optimal level of fluoride for a temperate climate was around 1 mg l^{-1}; this concentration was associated with a substantial resis-tance to tooth decay but with only a small and cosmetically insignificant increase in the prevalence of dental fluorosis.

Dental fluorosis is a cosmetic effect that ranges in appearance from scarcely discernible to a marked staining or pitting of the teeth in severe forms. It is caused by an elevated fluoride level in, or adjacent to, the developing enamel (Whitford, 1997). Thus, it follows that dental fluorosis can develop in children but not adults. Dental fluorosis in an adult is a result of high fluoride exposure when the adult was a child or adolescent. The problems involved in measuring the incidence and severity of dental fluorosis (USNRC, 1993) are beyond the scope of this work other than to note that adequately trained individuals are required. There are a variety of ways of describing dental fluorosis (USNRC, 1993) (see Appendix).

The first reports of the occurrence of dental fluorosis date back to 1888, when a family from Durango, Mexico were described as having "black teeth". Subsequently, erosion of dental enamel was described among inhabitants of Naples in 1891 and in Italian migrants to the USA from towns near Naples (Eager, 1901, cited by Belyakova and Zhavoronkov, 1978). Subsequently, dental fluorosis was described in the early 1900s at several locations in the USA (Black and McKay, 1916; Fleischer, 1962) and in many other countries around the world. Indeed, Belyakova and Zhavoronkov (1978) suggested that fluorosis might be one of the most widespread of endemic health problems associated with natural geochemistry.

Endemic fluorosis is now known to be global in scope, occurring on all continents and affecting many millions of people. Although no precise figures for the global number of persons affected are available, some figures at national levels have been given in the literature. Thus, for example, in China some 38 million people are reported to suffer from dental fluorosis and 1.7 million from the more severe skeletal fluorosis (WRI, 1990). In India, Susheela and Das (1988) suggested that around one million people suffer from serious and incapacitating skeletal fluorosis. Using the Chinese dental:skeletal fluorosis ratio, India could therefore have up to 20 million dental fluorosis sufferers, and in fact Mangla (1991) suggested that fluorosis affects an estimated 25 million people in India. Thus in India and China alone over 60 million people may be affected and, when other populations in Africa and the eastern Mediterranean in particular are taken into account, the global total may exceed 70 million.

3.3.2 *Skeletal effects*

Endemic skeletal fluorosis is well documented and is known to occur with a range of severity in several parts of the world, including India, China and northern, eastern, central and southern Africa. It is primarily associated with the consumption of drinking-water containing elevated levels of fluoride but exposure to additional sources of fluoride such as high fluoride coal is also potentially very important. This is compounded by a number of factors which include climate, related to water consumption, nutritional status and diet, including additional sources of fluoride and exposure to other substances that modify the absorption of fluoride into the body. Crippling skeletal fluorosis, which is associated with the higher levels of exposure, can result from osteosclerosis, ligamentous and tendinous calcification and extreme bone deformity. Evidence from occupational exposure also indicates that exposure to elevated concentrations of fluoride in the air may also be a cause of skeletal fluorosis (IPCS, 2002).

Although there are a large number of epidemiological studies available, the data are such that it is difficult to determine a clear exposure–response relationship. One possible feature of fluorosis is bone fracture, although some studies have reported a protective effect of fluoride on fracture. In an epidemiological study in China the relationship between fluoride intake via drinking-water and all other sources, and all fractures, followed a U shaped dose response with higher rates of fracture at very low intakes below 0.34 mg l^{-1} and high intakes above 4.32 mg l^{-1} (total intake 14 mg per day) (Li *et al.*, 2001). It was concluded by the IPCS that for a total intake of 14 mg per day there is a clear excess risk of skeletal adverse effects and there is suggestive evidence of an increased risk of effects on the skeleton at total fluoride intakes above about 6 mg per day (IPCS, 2002).

3.3.3 *Cancer*

Studies of occupationally exposed populations, primarily from aluminium smelting, have reported an increased incidence of, and mortality from, lung and bladder cancer and from cancers in other sites. However, the data are inconsistent and in a number of studies the results can be more readily attributed to exposure to other substances than fluoride. There have also been a significant number of epidemiological studies examining the possible association between various cancers and exposure to fluoride in drinking-water. However, in spite of the large number of studies conducted in a number of countries, there is no consistent evidence to demonstrate any association between the consumption of controlled fluoridated drinking-water and either morbidity or mortality from cancer (USPHS, 1991; USNRC, 1993; WHO, 1996; IPCS, 2002).

3.3.4 *Other possible health effects*

A number of epidemiological studies have been carried out to examine other possible adverse outcomes as a consequence of exposure to fluoride, either from drinking-water or as a consequence of occupation.

Studies on the association between exposure of mothers to fluoride in drinking-water and adverse pregnancy outcome have shown no increased risk of either spontaneous abortion or congenital malformations.

No reasonable evidence of effects on the respiratory, haematopoietic, hepatic or renal systems have emerged from studies of occupationally exposed populations that could be attributed specifically to fluoride exposure. In addition, such studies have failed to produce convincing evidence of genotoxic effects.

The majority of fluoride is excreted via the kidneys (USNRC, 1993). Thus it is reasonable that those with impaired renal function might be at greater risk of fluoride toxicity than those without. In discussing this point, WHO (1996) concluded that the data were too limited to permit any quantitative evaluation of possible increased sensitivity due to impaired kidney function.

3.3.5 *Acute effects*

A number of overdosing incidents have occurred, mostly in small water supplies, that practice artificial fluoridation. With well designed fail-safe equipment and working practices overdosing incidents can be avoided (Leland *et al.*, 1980). Where incidents of acute intoxication have been reported following overdosing in water supplies, fluoride levels have ranged from 30–1,000 mg l^{-1} (Peterson, 1988). To produce signs of acute fluoride intoxication, it is estimated that minimum oral doses of at least 1 mg fluoride per kg of body weight are required (WHO, 1996). Indeed, such doses could be expected from water with a fluoride content of approximately 30 mg l^{-1}.

3.4   References

Belyakova, T.M. and Zhavoronkov, A.A. 1978   A study of endemic fluorosis on the continents of the terrestrial globe. USSR Academy of Sciences. *Proceedings of the Biogeochemical Laboratory*, **15**, 37–53 (in Russian).

Black, G.V. and McKay, F.S. 1916 Mottled teeth: an endemic developmental imperfection of the enamel of the teeth heretofore unknown in the literature of dentistry. *Dent. Cosmos.*, **58**, 129–156.

Bucher, J.R., Hejtmancik, M.R., Todd, J.D. 2nd, Persing, R.L., Eustis, S.L. and Haseman, J.K. 1991 Results and conclusions of the National Toxicology Program's rodent carcinogenicity studies with sodium fluoride. *International Journal of Cancer*, **48**(5), 733–737.

Dean, H.T. 1942 The investigation of physiological effects by the epidemiological method. In: Moulton, R.F. [Ed] *Fluorine and Dental Health*. American Association for the Advancement of Science, Washington DC.

Edmunds, W.M. and Smedley, P.L. 1996 Groundwater geochemistry and health: an overview. In: Appleton, Fuge and McCall [Eds] *Environmental Geochemistry and Health*. Geological Society Special Publication No 113, 91–105.

IARC 1987 Overall evaluation of carcinogenicity: an updating of IARC monographs volumes 1–42. *IARC Monographs on the Evaluation of Carcinogenic Risks to Humans, Suppl. 7*. International Agency for Research on Cancer, Lyon, 208–210.

IPCS 2002 *Fluorides*. Environmental Health Criteria 227. World Health Organization, Geneva.

Leland, D.E., Powell, K.E. and Anderson, R.S. 1980 A fluoride overfeed incident at Harbour Springs, Mich., *Journal of the American Water Works Association*, **72**(4), 238–243.

Li, Y., Liang, C., Slemenda, C.W., Ji, R., Sun, S., Cao, J., Emsley, C,. Ma, F., Wu, Y., Ying, P., Zhang, Y., Gao, S., Zhang, W., Katz, B., Niu, S., Cao, S. and Johnston, C. 2001 Effect of long-term exposure to fluoride in drinking water on risks of bone fractures. *Journal of Bone Mineralisation Research*, **16**(5), 932–939.

Mangla, B. 1991 India's dentists squeeze fluoride warnings off tubes. *New Scientist*, **131**, 16.

Maurer, J., Chen, M., Boyson, B. and Anderson, R. 1990 Two-year carcinogenicity study of sodium fluoride in rats. *Journal of the National Cancer Institute*, **82**(13), 1118–1126.

Maurer, J., Chen, M., Boyson, B., Squire, R., Strandberg, J., Weisbrode, J. and Anderson, R. 1993 Confounded carcinogenicity study of sodium fluoride in CD-1 mice. *Regulatory Toxicology and Pharmacology*, **18**(2), 154–168.

NTP 1990 Toxicology and carcinogenesis studies with sodium fluoride (CAS No. 7681-49-4) in F344/N rats and B6C3F1 mice (drinking water studies). US Department of Health and Human Services, Public Health Service, National Institutes of Health, National Toxicology Programme (NTP TR 393), Research Triangle Park, North Carolina.

Peterson, L.R., Denis, D., Brown, H., Hadler, H. And Helgerston, S.D. 1988 Community health effects of a municipal water supply hyperfluoridation accident. *American Journal of Public Health*, **78**(6), 711–713.

Susheela, A.K. and Das, T.K. 1988 Fluoride toxicity and fluorosis: diagnostic test for early detection and preventive medicines adopted in India. [Abstract], International Symposium on Environmental Life Elements and Health, Beijing, 89.

USNRC 1993 *Health Effects of Ingested Fluoride*. US National Research Council, National Academy Press, Washington, D.C.

USPHS 1991 *PHS Review of Fluoride: Benefits and Risks: Report of Ad Hoc Subcommittee on Fluoride*. Committee to Co-ordinate Environmental Health and Related Programs. US Public Health Service.

Whitford, G.M. 1997 Determinants and mechanisms of enamel fluorosis. *Ciba Foundation Symposium*, **205**, 226–241.

WHO 1996 *Guidelines for Drinking-water Quality. Volume 2. Health Criteria and Other Supporting Information*. 2nd edition, World Health Organization, Geneva.

WRI (World Resources Institute) 1996 *World Resources, a Guide to the Global Environment: the Urban Environment*. WRI/UNEP/UNDP/WB, Oxford University Press.

4

Guidelines and standards

In 1984, WHO conducted an extensive review and found that there were insufficient data to conclude that fluoride produces cancer or birth defects. In addition,
WHO noted that mottling of teeth (i.e. dental fluorosis) is sometimes associated
with fluoride levels in drinking-water above 1.5 mg l^{-1} and crippling skeletal
fluorosis can ensue when fluoride levels exceed 10 mg l^{-1}. A guideline value of
1.5 mg l^{-1} was therefore recommended by WHO as a level at which dental
fluorosis should be minimal (WHO, 1984).

The 1.5 mg l^{-1} fluoride guideline value that was set in 1984 was subsequently
re-evaluated by WHO and it was concluded that there was no evidence to suggest
that it should be revized (WHO, 1996, 2004). The 1.5 mg l^{-1} guideline value of
WHO is not a "fixed" value but is intended to be adapted to take account of local
conditions (e.g. diet, water consumption, etc.).

4.1 Application of the WHO guideline value to local conditions

It is particularly important to consider climatic conditions, volume of water
intake and other factors when setting national standards for fluoride (WHO,
1996). This point is extremely important, not only when setting national standards for fluoride, but also when taking data from one part of the world and
applying them in regions where local conditions are significantly different.

The effects of fluoride are best predicted by the dose (i.e. mg fluoride per kg of body weight per day), the duration of exposure and other factors such as age (e.g. dental fluorosis). However, most epidemiological studies concerning the effects of fluoride on teeth and bone have correlated the effects with the concentration of fluoride in the drinking-water (mg l^{-1} fluoride) consumed rather than total fluoride exposure.

Provided water is the major source of fluoride exposure, and water consumption is reasonably constant in the population examined, the concentration of fluoride in mg l^{-1} is a reasonable surrogate for fluoride exposure in that population. However, populations that drink significantly different volumes of water per day containing the same level of fluoride are exposed to significantly different daily doses of fluoride. Because the daily fluoride dose determines the likely health outcome, data obtained from, for example, temperate climates are not directly applicable to hot humid regions where significantly more water is consumed.

Ideally, epidemiological data for fluoride should be extrapolated from one region to another on the basis of mg fluoride per kg body weight per day. At a minimum, daily water consumption data in several regions would be needed for this. However, water consumption data are typically only available for a few countries in temperate climates, such as Canada (Environmental Health Directorate, 1977), USA (Ershow and Cantor, 1989) and UK (Hopkin and Ellis, 1980).

While water is frequently the major source of fluoride exposure, this is not always the case as exposure from the diet and from air can be important in some situations (see section 2.2). There is also a clear indication that high altitudes can increase fluoride retention and have an effect on dental appearance independent of fluoride exposure (Whitford, 1997). While the world-wide significance of this effect is not clear at present, it does appear to be a local factor that needs to be considered in some situations (Cao et al., 1997).

Thus, although it is particularly important to consider climatic conditions, volumes of water intake, diet and other factors when considering fluoride (WHO, 1996), it is not clear how many of these local conditions can be applied quantitatively, because of a lack of data.

Perhaps the best general advice that can be given in relation to local conditions is that, at a minimum, the fluoride level in local water supplies should be monitored and the population examined for signs of excessive fluoride exposure (e.g. moderate and/or severe dental fluorosis and crippling skeletal fluorosis).

Where treatment to remove fluoride is practised, chemicals used should be of a grade suitable for use in drinking-water supply as outlined in the WHO Guidelines for Drinking-water Quality.

4.2 References

Cao, J., Bai, X., Zhao, Y., Zhou, D., Fang, S., Jia, M. and Wu, J. 1997 Brick tea consumption as the cause of dental fluorosis among children from Mongol, Kazak and Yugu populations in China. *Food and Chemical Toxicology*, **35**(8), 827–833.

Environmental Health Directorate 1977 *Tap Water Consumption in Canada*. 77-EHD-18, Ministry of Health and Welfare.

Ershow, A.G. and Cantor, K.P. 1989 *Total Water and Tapwater Intake in the United States: Population-Based Estimates of Quantities and Sources*. No. 263-MD-810264, National Cancer Institute.

Hopkin, S.M. and Ellis, J.C. 1980 *Drinking Water Consumption in Great Britain*. Technical Report TR 137, Water Research Centre, Medmenham, UK.

Whitford, G.M. 1997 Determinants and mechanisms of enamel fluorosis. *Ciba Foundation Symposium*, **205**, 226–241.

WHO 1984 *Guidelines for Drinking-water Quality. Volume 2. Health Criteria and Other Supporting Information*. World Health Organization, Geneva.

WHO 1996 *Guidelines for Drinking-water Quality. Volume 2. Health Criteria and Other Supporting* Information. 2nd edition. World Health Organization, Geneva.

WHO 2004 *Guidelines for Drinking-water Quality. Volume 1. Recommendations*. 3rd edition. World Health Organization, Geneva.

5

Removal of excessive fluoride

Occurrence of fluoride at excessive levels in drinking-water in developing countries is a serious problem. Its detection demands analytical grade chemicals and laboratory equipment and skills. Similarly, the prevention of fluorosis through management of drinking-water is a difficult task, which requires favourable conditions combining knowledge, motivation, prioritization, discipline and technical and organizational support. Many filter media and several water treatment methods are known to remove fluoride from water. However, many initiatives on defluoridation of water have resulted in frustration and failure (COWI, 1998). Therefore, in any attempt to mitigate fluoride contamination for an affected community, the provision of safe, low fluoride water from alternative sources, either as an alternative source or for blending, should be investigated as the first option.

In cases where alternative sources are not available, defluoridation of water is the only measure remaining to prevent fluorosis (Figure 5.1). However, there are several different defluoridation methods. What may work in one community may not work in another. What may be appropriate at a certain time and stage of urbanization, may not be at another. It is therefore most important to select an appropriate defluoridation method carefully if a sustainable solution to a fluorosis problem is to be achieved (Figure 5.2).

This chapter introduces the basic characterization of the removal methods, followed by discussion of the most promising defluoridation methods; bone

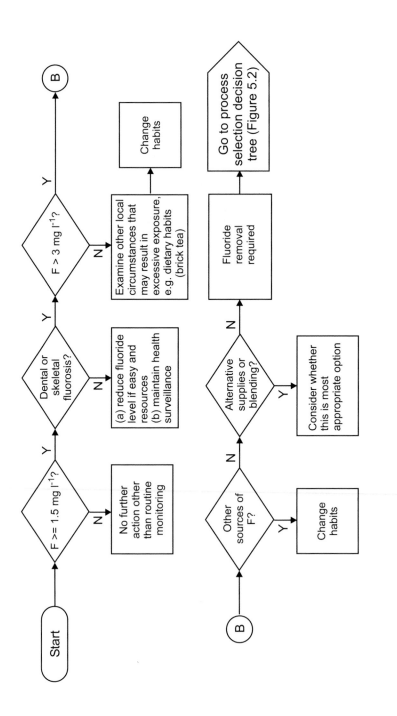

Figure 5.1 Decision tree for appropriate action in relation to elevated concentrations of fluoride in water sources.

Potentially available and acceptable processes and materials:

Bone charcoal (BC); Contact precipitation (CP); Clay (CL); Activated alumina (AA);
Calcium chloride (CC); Monosodium phosphate (MP); Nalgonda (NA)

Note:

*"**Available**"* means **locally available** with continuity of **supply** and **affordable**.
*"**Acceptable**"* means that the society accepts use of the material in question.

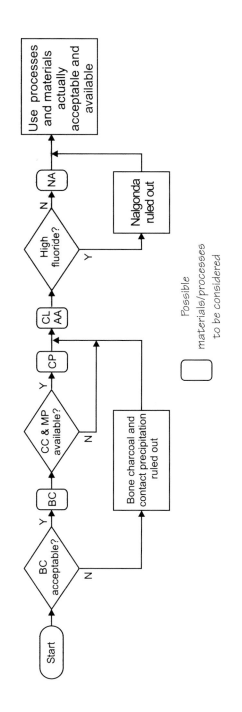

Figure 5.2   Process selection decision tree.

charcoal, contact precipitation, Nalgonda, activated alumina and clay. Finally the methods discussed are compared using indicators, which may be appropriate in developing countries.

Advanced treatment technologies, e.g. reverse osmosis, electrodialysis and distillation, plus methods based on patented media and natural media of restricted interest are largely excluded from the scope of this document. Defluoridation of drinking-water is technically feasible at point-of-use (at the tap), for small communities of users (e.g. wellhead application) and for large drinking-water supplies. Activated alumina and reverse osmosis are the most common technologies. Activated alumina can concurrently remove other anions, such as arsenate. Reverse osmosis achieves significant removal of virtually all dissolved contaminants.

Point-of-use systems can produce sufficient quantities of treated water for drinking and cooking requirements of several persons. Numerous plumbed-in, small distillation units are marketed that have been tested and can produce several gallons per day or much larger volumes. Many certified low pressure reverse osmosis units are available with rated capacities in the range of 8–33 gallons per day. Point-of-use defluoridation using activated alumina anion exchange is capable of removing fluoride from small volumes of water, but international performance standards have not been developed to date.

Community-sized, commercially available, package water treatment systems that use activated alumina or reverse osmosis technology also exist. They can be purchased as a complete unit that can be readily shipped and installed on-site. These can produce hundreds of gallons or more of treated, low fluoride water per day. Large defluoridation systems can also be designed and constructed on-site to engineer's specifications (Heidewiller, 1990; Bulusu *et al.*, 1993).

5.1   Method characterization

5.1.1 Scale and decentralization

Conventional water treatment, as carried out in both rural and urban areas in industrialized countries, takes place typically:

- in a water works without direct involvement of the users,
- under the supervision of skilled operators, and
- where the affordability of treatment is taken for granted.

In such cases the method of treatment is well established and well controlled. However, it requires major input of resources and may have serious limitations or disadvantages in less-developed countries, especially in rural areas where the water users are scattered or the supply is entirely local. Here treatment may only

Table 5.1   Differences in characterization of water treatment methods in conventional systems as taking place in industrialized and developing countries.

Criteria	Industrialized countries	Developing countries
Set-up and water flow	Always continuous, often in columns	Often discontinuous in columns Fill and draw in batch
Scale and treatment site	Always at water works, usually close to water source	At water works At village community level At household level
Treatment media/process	Contact precipitation Activated alumina Synthetic resins Reverse osmosis Electrodialysis	Bone charcoal Contact precipitation Nalgonda Activated alumina Clay Other naturally occurring media

be feasible at a decentralized level, e.g. at community village level or at household level (Table 5.1).

5.1.2 Set-up and flow

Water treatment design should account for the required storage of water and different feed and withdrawal patterns. Filter columns, as used for bone charcoal, activated alumina and clay, are often fed intermittently and operate at various flow rates. Thus there will be a need for a pre-storage container and a control of the flow rate in order to ensure a minimum contact time. Batch units, as in the Nalgonda technique, are often fed once a day. In both cases a separate clean water container would be useful or even essential.

Even in situations where the water is supplied through piped schemes, the decentralized solution may be more advantageous. This is because there is no need to remove the fluoride from the water that is not consumed, i.e. used for cooking or drinking, and water demand for all uses is often more than 10 times the water needed for drinking and cooking. Defluoridation of the total amount of water used would, therefore, be more costly, and possibly unaffordable for the community or the household. Unnecessary removal of fluoride from water would result in accumulation of unnecessarily large amounts of toxic sludge, which is likely to create an environmental disposal problem.

Whilst water supply in industrialized countries is typically stable and continuous through household connections; arrangements in developing countries may be more variable and include piped systems, community source treatment and/or household treatment. For example, the bone charcoal process can be utilized in water works, in a village plant and at the household level. Also it can be used in columns for continuous supply or in batches, e.g. water buckets.

Taking into consideration the environmental and socio-economic sustainability of the treatment system, the difference between a centralized system and a household system may be much more significant than the difference between bone charcoal and alumina.

5.1.3 Media and process

Defluoridation processes can be categorized into three main groups:

- Bone charcoal, activated alumina and clay resemble *sorption media*, preferably to be packed in columns to be used for a period of operation. Sorption processes result in saturated columns to be renewed or regenerated.
- Aluminium sulfate and lime in the Nalgonda technique, polyaluminium chloride, lime and similar compounds act as *co-precipitation chemicals* to be added daily and in batches. Precipitation techniques produce a certain amount of sludge every day.
- Calcium and phosphate compounds are the so-called *contact precipitation chemicals* to be added to the water upstream of a catalytic filter bed. In contact precipitation there is no sludge and no saturation of the bed, only the accumulation of the precipitate in the bed.

Magnesite, apophyllite, natrolite, stilbite, clinoptilolite, gibbsite, goethite, kaolinite, halloysite, bentonite, vermiculite, zeolite(s), serpentine, alkaline soil, acidic clay, kaolinitic clay, China clay, aiken soil, Fuller's earth, diatomaceous earth and Ando soil are among the numerous naturally occurring minerals which have been studied and confirmed to adsorb fluoride from water (Bower and Hatcher, 1967; Maruthamuthu and Sivasamy, 1994; Bjorvartn and Bårdsen, 1997; Singano et al., 1997). The common feature of these minerals is their contents of metal lattice hydroxyl-groups, which can be exchanged with fluoride. Ion exchange of a metal compound M:

$$M\text{-}OH_{(s)} + F^- \quad M\text{-}F_{(s)} + OH^- \tag{1}$$

In general, the minerals themselves do have some capacity for fluoride removal. The capacity can be increased through "activation" by acid washing, calcination or air drying. None of these minerals can be considered to be a universal defluoridation agent. Should one of them, however, occur adjacent to a fluorotic area, and thus be available at low or no cost, it may be considered as the medium of choice for that particular area. In this document clay is used as a prototype for these minerals. Clay, for example, has been reported to be appropriate for use in Sri Lanka (Padmasiri, 1998).

5.2   Bone charcoal

5.2.1 Description

Bone charcoal is a blackish, porous, granular material. The major components of bone charcoal are calcium phosphate 57–80 per cent, calcium carbonate 6–10 per cent, and activated carbon 7–10 per cent. In contact with water the bone charcoal is able, to a limited extent, to absorb a wide range of pollutants such as colour, taste and odour components. Moreover, bone charcoal has the specific ability to take up fluoride from water. This is believed to be due to its chemical composition, mainly as hydroxyapatite, $Ca_{10}(PO_4)_6(OH)_2$, where one or both the hydroxyl-groups can be replaced with fluoride. The principal reaction is hydroxyl-fluoride exchange of apatite:

$$Ca_{10}(PO_4)_6(OH)_2 + 2F^- Ca_{10}(PO_4)_6 F_2 + 2 OH^- \qquad (2)$$

5.2.2 Preparation

The preparation of bone charcoal is crucial to optimize its properties as a defluoridation agent and as a water purifier. Unless carried out properly, the bone charring process may result in a product of low defluoridation capacity and/or a deterioration in water quality. Water treated with poor bone charcoal may taste and smell like rotten meat and be aesthetically unacceptable. Once consumers are exposed to such a smell or taste, they may reject the bone charcoal treatment process and it may be difficult to persuade them to try water from the process again. It is therefore essential to ensure that the bone charcoal quality is always good. Even single failures in the production may be disastrous for a defluoridation project (Dahi and Bregnhøj, 1997).

Another potential disadvantage of bone charcoal is related to the problems of supply to local users. Industrially prepared bone charcoal used to be commercially widely available some decades ago. Today the commercial distribution of bone charcoal is much more limited. One option may therefore be to prepare the bone charcoal at village factory or household level (Jacobsen and Dahi, 1998).

Bone charcoal is prepared by heating ground bone in retorts or in pots stacked in a furnace resembling a potter's kiln, without or with only limited admission of atmospheric oxygen. Ground bone is prepared industrially by degreasing, boiling, washing and drying, prior to grinding and sifting out. The bone grains are normally available from the manufacturing of bone meal used as fodder additive (Mantell, 1968). Several attempts to find optimum heating temperature and

Table 5.2   Critical parameters for bone charcoal preparation and quality testing.

Quality criteria	Properties		Reason for low quality
	Appropriate quality	Poor quality	
Bone charcoal grains:			
Defluoridation capacity	>4 mg g^{-1}	<3 mg g^{-1}	Charring: temp. >550 °C +oxidation
Residual organics	Undetectable	Detectable	Charring: low temp./short duration
Carbon content	6–10%	<6%	Charring: oxidation
Grain size, mm	1–3	<1 or >3	Raw crushing, insufficient sorting
Non-uniformity	Low	High	Insufficient sorting
Colour	Black	Grey-White	Charring: temp. >550 °C +oxidation
BET (m^2 g^{-1})[a]	120–150	<100	Charring: temp. >550 °C +oxidation
Equilibrium water:			
Taste	Tasteless	Unpleasant	Insufficient charring/overdose
Smell	No smell	Unpleasant	Insufficient charring/overdose
Colour	Colourless	Yellowish	Insufficient charring/overdose
pH	7.5–8.5	>8.5	Charring: temp. >550 °C +oxidation
Alkalinity	<1 meq l^{-1}	>1 meq l^{-1}	Charring: temp. >550 °C +oxidation

[a]   BET is the Brunauer, Emmett and Teller index for specific surface area determination
        using nitrogen (m^2 g^{-1})
Source: Dahi and Bregnhøj (1997)

duration seem to have failed. Heating to 550 °C for about 4 hours or even less is in principle sufficient, but the process in total, including heating up and cooling down, would take not less than 24 hours. The required temperature and duration of heating would be expected to depend to a large extent on the batch size and the packing rather than the type or the nature of the bone.

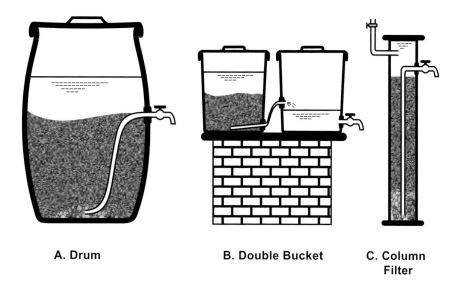

| A. Drum | B. Double Bucket | C. Column Filter |

Figure 5.3   Three most common domestic units for sorption defluoridation.

At village level the process can be carried out in a kiln, in which the raw bones can be packed directly along with coal. This technique has an advantage, because crushing of the charred bone is much less labourious than uncharred bones. Table 5.2 illustrates that poor bone charcoal quality would mainly be due to:

- Insufficient charring, i.e. temperature too low and duration too short.
- Admission of oxygen, i.e. running the process as calcination instead of charring.
- Overheating of the bones, especially if oxygen is admitted to the heated bone material.
- Inhomogeneous heating which always results in poor bone charcoal quality.

It must be noted that the preparation of bone charcoal may, if not carried out in a properly designed kiln or furnace, cause an extremely unpleasant smell even in a spacious rural environment (Jacobsen and Dahi, 1998).

5.2.3 Technical configuration

Figure 5.3 illustrates the three most common types of domestic bone charcoal filters and Table 5.3 indicates the differences between them. The illustrated technical configurations are commonly used for all types of sorption process.

Table 5.3 Comparison of the three types of domestic bone charcoal filters illustrated in Figure 5.3.

	Drum	Double bucket	Column
Advantages:			
No daily dosage of chemicals	Yes	Yes	Yes
Theoretical medium capacity can be fully utilized	No	No	Yes
High removal efficiency can be ensured; minimum short circuiting	No	No	Yes
Easy to construct, even by the users	Yes	Yes	Variable
Construction materials are cheap and widely available	Yes	Yes	Variable
Can be sized for one or several families or groups, e.g. a school	Yes	No	Yes
Can be connected to an overhead raw water reservoir (tight cover)	Yes	No	Yes
Can be connected to piped water supply (non return valve)	Variable	No	Yes
Can be made of normal water buckets or purchased ready-made	Variable	Yes	No
Disadvantages:			
Medium needs renewal or regeneration when saturated	Yes	Yes	Yes
Saturation point difficult to predict; requires monitoring	Yes	Yes	Yes
Low removal efficiency if water is withdrawn at high rate	Yes	Yes	No
Risk of water drainage from the medium, "drying"	No	Variable	No
Less convenient packing and setting up	No	No	Variable

One of the differences concerns the water flow in the filter. In the column filter the flow resembles *plug flow*, where the upper parts of the filter bed become saturated at a time where the lower parts are still fresh. Then the saturation zone moves slowly towards the bottom effluent point. This kind of flow allows for saturation of the medium with respect to the high fluoride raw water, hence the high capacity utilization in the column systems. In the drum or the bucket filter the flow resembles a totally mixed system, where the medium at saturation point is in equilibrium with the treated water. Hence the low capacity utilization in the drum and the bucket type filters.

Another difference between the various configurations is whether the filter allows the filter medium to drain water, if treated water is withdrawn without ensuring an adequate influent, allowing the medium to become dry. "Drying" the medium results in disturbance of the sorption process and more contact time would be required to re-establish treatment. Unfortunately this point is over-looked in many household filter designs.

5.2.4 *Regeneration*

It is feasible to regenerate bone charcoal saturated with fluoride by allowing equilibrium with 1 per cent solution of sodium hydroxide followed by washing or neutralization of the surplus caustic soda (AWWA, 1971). Regeneration is probably only cost effective at a large-scale water works level or in the case of a shortage of the medium. At village-community and household levels, it may be environmentally acceptable to use the saturated bone charcoal as a fertilizer and soil conditioner.

5.2.5 *Design criteria*

Apart from the daily water demand (the load), and the raw water fluoride concentration, the key parameter of all designs would be the bone charcoal theoretical defluoridation capacity (Γ). This is expressed as the amount of fluoride absorbed by one grain of bone charcoal at saturation. Unfortunately, in laboratory studies Γ is often estimated with respect to unrealistically high fluoride concentrations. In water treatment the operational defluoridation capacity should be used, with reference to the given fluoride concentration and experimental set-up. Obviously, saturation with respect to the raw water fluoride concentration, as in column filters, would result in much more efficient utilization of a bone charcoal medium than saturation with respect to the effluent concentration at the end of a filter period, as in bucket filters (drum or bucket filters).

Thus at an operational level, Γ depends on the loading pattern, i.e. the variation of water flow through the filter medium, and the *back mix* pattern, i.e. to what extent the water flow resembles a *plug flow* through the filter medium. Different sorption models have been developed to simulate the operation of bone

charcoal filters and thus to create a rational background for the design of these
filters (Dahi and Bregnhøj, 1997).

Examples of the design of bone charcoal filters are given in Table 5.4.
Assuming the theoretical bone charcoal defluoridation capacity is 6 mg g^{-1}, the
operational capacity would then be 4 mg g^{-1} for column filters and 2 mg g^{-1} for
bucket filters. It can generally be assumed that:

- Operational defluoridation capacity in column filters $\cong$ 2/3 theoretical
  defluoridation capacity
- Operational defluoridation capacity in bucket filters $\cong$ 1/3 theoretical
  defluoridation capacity

Table 5.4 demonstrates how the dosage equivalent is 2 and 4 g l^{-1} respectively for column filter and bucket and drum filters. If the same dose is added, as
in a batch process, the residual concentration from a column filter will be lower.

5.2.6 Cost

All three types of bone charcoal filters can be made locally using cheap, locally
available, robust and corrosion resistant materials such as plastic, concrete,
ferrocement or galvanized iron sheets. In such cases the unit price would be
affordable to most motivated communities.

The price of bone charcoal on the other hand may be significant, depending
on the method of manufacture. For example, in 1995 quotations were collected
for large scale delivery of bone charcoal *ab fabric* from UK, China and the
United Republic of Tanzania. The prices given were US\$ 2280, US\$ 333 and
US\$ 167 per ton respectively. Finally, it was discovered that the bone charcoal
could be prepared in a low cost, locally-made kiln from freely-collected bones in
the Arusha region in the United Republic of Tanzania by using about 120 kg of
charcoal per tonne of bone.

5.2.7 Experience

Bone charcoal is the oldest known water defluoridation agent. It was used in USA
in the 1940s through to the 1960s, when bone charcoal was commercially widely
available because of its large scale use in the sugar industry (AWWA, 1971).

The first domestic defluoridators were developed in the early 1960s as column
filters similar to the one shown in Figure 5.3 (Dunckley and Malthus, 1961; Roche
1964). In 1988 the ICOH filter type was launched by WHO (Phantumvanit *et al.*,
1988) and has since been tested both in and outside Thailand. In contrast to the
filter described by Roche (1964), the ICOH type filter is enriched with charcoal,
and thus has the capacity for removal of impurities in case of either poor raw
water quality or insufficient bone charring. Furthermore, the water flow in the
ICOH defluoridator occurs by siphoning the raw water from an overhead

container. This arrangement allows for manual adjustment of the water flow by using tube clamps, but the unit would need supervision and operator training in order to avoid the column running dry or the clean water jar overflowing.

Today bone charcoal defluoridation at waterworks has been replaced by the use of ion-exchange resins and activated alumina. At a domestic level, bone charcoal defluoridation seems to work well in Thailand and Africa, but so far there is no experience of wide scale implementation.

Relatively expensive filters are commercially available based on packages of medium and a modification of the candle-type stainless steel domestic filters.

5.2.8 Local customs and beliefs

One of the constraints of bone charcoal defluoridation is related to religious beliefs in some societies and communities that any use of animal bones is unacceptable. In such cases the use of bone charcoal must be avoided.

However, this may relate only to the use of bone charcoal originating from certain animals, such as cows among Hindus, pigs among Muslims and Jews, and hyena and dogs among many Africans. From a scientific point of view all types of bones are equally good as raw materials for bone charcoal, but in such circumstances the problem would be solved through production of bone charcoal in accordance with local acceptability and ensuring that this is widely known in the community.

Irrespective of local beliefs, microbiological, aesthetic and psychological problems would render bone charcoal defluoridation completely unacceptable, if drinking-water was allowed to percolate through a medium containing organic residues from animals. It must, therefore, be emphasized that this could only happen in the case of incomplete charring. Properly prepared bone charcoal is totally mineralized and, if this is the case, the black colour of the product shows that it is only non-organic activated carbon.

5.3 Contact precipitation

5.3.1 Description

Contact precipitation is a technique by which fluoride is removed from the water through addition of calcium and phosphate compounds and then bringing the water in contact with an already saturated bone charcoal medium. In solutions containing calcium, phosphate and fluoride, the precipitation of calcium fluoride and/or fluorapatite is theoretically feasible, but practically impossible due to slow reaction kinetics. It has recently been reported that the precipitation is easily catalysed in a contact bed that acts as a filter for the precipitate (Dahi, 1996). Using

Table 5.4 Examples of design of the bone charcoal filters illustrated in Figure 5.3. For simplification the filters are designed assuming the same daily water consumption, raw water and bone charcoal quality.

Parameters:		Unit	Design examples		
			Drum type	Bucket type	Column type
Given:					
D	Daily personal water demand	$l/(c \times d)$	3	3	3
N	Number of users	p	6	6	6
OP	Operation period	months	12	3	6
Γ_o	Operational sorption capacity	$g\ kg^{-1}$	2	2	4
σ	Bulk density of medium	$kg\ l^{-1}$	0.83	0.83	0.83
F_i	Raw water fluoride concentration	$mg\ l^{-1}$	10	10	10
F_t	Treated water average fluoride concentration	$mg\ l^{-1}$	1	1	1
$VR_{SW/M}$	Volume ratio supernatant water/medium	–	2	2.5	0.2
$VR_{CW/M}$	Volume ratio clean water container/medium	–	0	3.5	0
Derived:					
$Q = D \times N$	Daily water treatment	l/d	18	18	18
$V_T = OP \times Q$	Total volume of water treated in a filter period	l	6,500	1,600	3,200
$F_T = V_T \times (Fi - F_t)/1{,}000$	Total fluoride removal during a period	g	60	15	30
$M = F_T / \Gamma_o$	Amount of medium required for renewal	kg	30	7	7
$V_M = M / \sigma$	Volume of medium in the filter	l	35	9	9

Continued

Table 5.4 Continued

Parameters:	Unit	Design examples		
		Drum type	Bucket type	Column type
Derived cont.:				
$BV = VT / V_M$ Number of bed volumes treated in a filter period	–	185	185	370
$V_{SW} = VR_{SW/M} / V_M$				
Volume capacity of supernatant water	l	70	22	2
$V_{CW} = VR_{CW/M} / V_M$				
Volume capacity of clean water container	l	0	31	0
$V_F = V_M + V_{SW} + V_{CW}$				
Total volume of filter	l	105	62	11
Corresponding dimensions:				
Ø Filter diameter (selected as available)	cm	42	32	12
$H_F = V_F / (\pi \times (Ø/2)^2)$				
Total height of the filter	cm	75	75	92

calcium chloride (CC) and sodium dihydrogenphosphate (MSP) or "monosodium phosphate" as chemicals, the following equations illustrate the removal:

Dissolution of CC:
$$CaCl_2\ 2H_2O\ (s) = Ca^{2+} + 2\ Cl^- + 2H_2O \tag{3}$$

Dissolution of MSP:
$$NaH_2PO_4\ H_2O\ (s) = PO_4^{3-} + Na^+ + 2\ H^+ + H_2O \tag{4}$$

Precipitation of calcium fluoride:
$$Ca^{2+} + 2\ F^- = CaF_{2(s)} \tag{5}$$

Precipitation of fluorapatite:
$$10\ Ca^{2+} + 6\ PO_4^- + 2\ F^- = Ca_{10}(PO_4)_6\ F_{2(s)} \tag{6}$$

The plants comprise a column, containing a relatively small, saturated bone charcoal contact bed. Gravel, or coarse grained bone charcoal, is used as a supporting medium. Above the bed a relatively large space is used for mixing the chemical with the raw water. From the bed the defluoridated water flows continuously by gravity to a shallow, but wide, clean water tank. One or more clean water taps are fitted at the bottom. The flow from the raw water tank to the clean water tank is constrained by a valve or a narrow tube arrangement to allow for appropriate contact time in the bed. Too short contact time would reduce the removal capacity and increase the escape of chemicals in the treated water. Too long contact time may result in precipitation of calcium phosphates in the upper parts of the filter bed, thus also reducing the removal efficiency. The optimum contact time is not yet known but contact times of 20 to 30 minutes have been shown to produce excellent operation. The filter resistance is negligible compared to the flow resistance through the tube and/or the valve (Dahi, 1998). The process seems to be promising, because it implies:
- relatively low daily working load;
- high reliability without the need of surveillance of flow or effluent concentration;
- high removal efficiency, even in case of high raw water concentrations;
- low operating cost; and
- no health risk in the case of misuse or over-dosage of chemicals.

5.3.2 Technical configuration

Although it has so far only been implemented at village level in the United Republic of Tanzania and in Kenya, contact precipitation is probably suitable for implementation at any required level. Figures 5.4 and 5.5 show contact

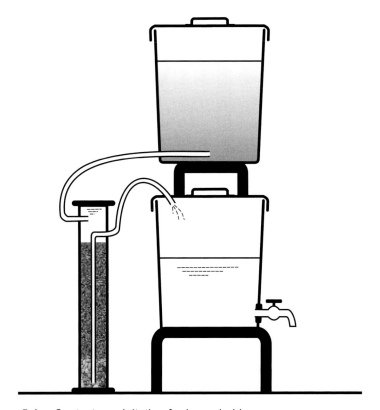

Figure 5.4   Contact precipitation for household use.

precipitation plant as developed for household use and installed at various schools in the rural areas of the Arusha region, the Un ited Republic of Tanzania.

In a large scale plant both the contact bed and the defluoridated water tank may be supplied with plastic tubes used as manometers. The ends of both tubes are located a few centimetres below the upper edges of the tanks to avoid overflow.

Chemicals in stock solutions

Any calcium and phosphate compounds can be used. It is, however, important to dissolve the chemicals prior to mixing with the water. As a calcium compound, calcium chloride (CC) may be used. As a phosphate compound, sodium dihydrogenphosphate (also called monosodium phosphate or MSP) may be used. Both compounds are easily dissolved, quite cheap and widely used. Calcium chloride is manufactured as technical grade flakes containing 77–80 per cent calcium chloride. One MSP product is fabricated as a granulated formulation

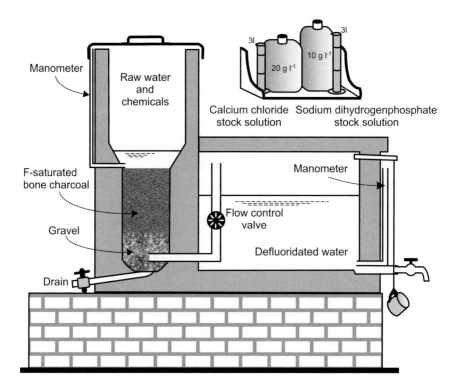

Figure 5.5   Contact precipitation of fluoride as invented in Ngurdoto. After Dahi, 1998.

containing 24 per cent phosphorus and 20 per cent sodium. The bulk density of the chemicals may be 1.04 for CC and 0.95 for MSP.

The chemicals are preferably prepared as stock solutions to be used in aliquots. The two stock solutions may be prepared once every month, for example, but should not be mixed before treatment in order to avoid the precipitation of calcium phosphate. Two special measuring cups may be used for volumetric portioning of the chemicals. It is advisable to check the bulk density as it may vary for different brands. The stock solutions, stored in Jerry cans, along with the respective chemical bags and the measuring cups and cylinders may be coloured respectively red and green in order to minimize the risk of exchange and so incorrect dosage.

Operation of the domestic unit

Initially the raw water bucket would be empty. The plant operator starts by closing the flow control valve completely and one and a half litres of each of the stock solutions are added to be mixed with a part of the raw water brought to the raw water compartment. As the remaining raw water is poured into the raw water compartment, the supernatant water is completely mixed. The flow control valve is then opened, but only to allow a slow flow through the contact bed, the average filtration velocity not exceeding 0.5 m per hour.

Operation of the community plant

Initially the raw water column would be empty. The plant operator starts by closing the flow control valve completely and each of the two stock solution aliquots are added to be mixed with a part of the raw water brought to the raw water compartment. As the remaining raw water is filled into the raw water compartment, the supernatant water would be completely mixed. The flow control valve is then opened, but only to allow a slow flow through the contact bed, the average filtration velocity not exceeding 0.5 m per hour or about 0.5 cm per minute.

5.3.3 Design criteria

The construction of the contact precipitation plants is simple, but the theoretical background for doing it is not. Probably both reactions (5) and (6) play important roles, but the extent to which each reaction occurs is not well understood. In calcium fluoride precipitation, the Ca/F weight ratio is about 1, equivalent to a CC/F ratio of about 4. In fluorapatite precipitation, the Ca/F is 11 and the PO_4/F ratio is 15, equivalent to a CC/F ratio of about 39 and a MSP/F ratio of about 23.

Thus the more fluoride that is precipitated as calcium fluoride, rather than as fluorapatite, the lower is the required dosage of chemicals. Calcium fluoride precipitation is probably more dominant with higher raw water fluoride concentration. Long term operation of the contact precipitation technique in the United Republic of Tanzania, where the fluoride concentration is about 10 mg l^{-1}, has shown that the process functions effectively when the dosage ratios are 30 and 15 for CC and MSP respectively. This dosage would ensure at least 65 per cent precipitation of fluorapatite and a surplus of calcium for precipitation of the residual fluoride as calcium fluoride. This dosage is shown in Table 5.5. Over-dosage is of no economic or health significance and lower dosage levels may be recommended on a trial and error basis.

Table 5.5 Examples of design of domestic bucket and school brick-built plants for contact precipitation of fluoride.[a]

Parameters		Unit	Design examples	
			Domestic	School/Market
Given				
D	Daily personal water demand	$l/(c \times d)$	3	0.5
N	Number of users	p	6	500
F_i	Raw water fluoride concentration	$mg\ l^{-1}$	10	10
F_t	Treated water average fluoride concentration	$mg\ l^{-1}$	0.4	0.4
ε	Medium porosity	–	0.56	0.56
σ	Medium bulk density	$kg\ l^{-1}$	0.83	0.83
v	Filtration velocity	m/h	0.5	0.5
t_c	Contact time $(=H_c \times \varepsilon/v)$	h	0.3	0.3
t_F	Filtration time $(=Q/v \times \pi \times (Ø/2)^2))$	h	4	4
$VR_{RW/Q}$	Volume ratio raw water/daily water treated	–	1.1	1.2
$VR_{BC/Q}$	Volume bone charcoal medium/daily water treated	–	0.3	0.3
$VR_{CW/Q}$	Volume bone charcoal medium/daily water treated	–	1.1	2
$MR_{CC/F}$	Mass ratio calcium chloride/daily fluoride loading	–	30	30
$MR_{MSP/F}$	Mass ratio MSP/daily fluoride loading	–	15	15

Continued

Table 5.5 Continued

Parameters		Unit	Design examples	
			Domestic	School/Market
Derived:				
$Q = D \times N$	Daily water treatment	l/d	18	250
$F_T = Q \times F_i / 1{,}000$	Total daily fluoride loading ($\approx$ removal)	g/d	0.18	2.5
$\varnothing_{BC} = 2(Q/(t_F \times v \times \pi)^{0.5})$	Diameter of contact bed	cm	11	40
$H_{BC} = t_C \times v/\varepsilon$	Height of contact bed (medium only)	cm	27	40
$M_{CC} = F_T \times WR_{CC/F}$	Total daily dosage of CC	g/d	5	75
$M_{MSP} = F_T \times MR_{MSP/F}$	Total daily dosage of MSP	g/d	3	40
$V_{RW} = Q \times VR_{CW/Q}$	Volume of raw water bucket/column	l	20	300
$V_{BC} = Q \times VR_{BC/Q}$	Volume of contact bed medium	l	2.4	33.5
$M_{BC} = V_{BC} \times \sigma$	Mass of contact bed medium	kg	2	30
$V_{CW} = Q \times VR_{CW/Q}$	Volume of clean water bucket/tank	l	20	500
$W_{RW} \approx (V_{RW})^{1/3}$	Width of raw water column	cm	–	65
$L_{RW} \approx W_{RW}$	Length of raw water column	cm	–	65
$H_{RW} = V_{RW} / (W_{RW} \times L_{RW})$	Height of raw water column	cm	–	70
$\varnothing_{CB} = \varnothing_{BC}$	Diameter of contact bed compartment	cm	–	40
$H_{CB} = H_{CW}$	Height of contact bed compartment	cm	–	65
$W_{CW} = W_{RW}$	Width of clean water tank	cm	–	65
$H_{CW} = H_{CB}$	Height of clean water tank	cm	–	65
$L_{CW} = V_{CW} / (B_{CW} \times H_{CW})$	Length of clean water tank	cm	–	120

[a] It is assumed that the calcium compound (CC) used is calcium chloride containing about 27% calcium, and sodium dihydrogenphosphate (MSP) containing about 65% phosphate.

5.3.4 Cost

Quotations were obtained in 1996 for calcium chloride and sodium dihydrogen-phosphate wholesale. The figures given were US$ 283 and US$ 780 per ton respectively.

5.3.5 Experience

Experience from the Arusha region of the United Republic of Tanzania has shown that construction of a plant needs skilled supervision, at least until a team of bricklayers has completed the construction of a few plants. The critical points seem to be:

- watertight cement or plastic plastering;
- proper installation of fittings; and
- adjustment of the flow rate to meet the requirements of contact time and filtration time.

Once these issues are addressed, it has been demonstrated that a young school pupil can easily operate the plant satisfactorily. No bacterial growth or disturbance in the efficiency of the plant has been observed during stagnation during a rainy season or a summer vacation.

5.4   Nalgonda

5.4.1 Description

The Nalgonda process was adapted and developed in India by the National Environmental Engineering Research Institute (NEERI) and developed to be used at both the community or household levels. The process is aluminium sulfate based coagulation-flocculation sedimentation, where the dosage is designed to ensure fluoride removal from the water. Aluminium sulfate, $Al_2 (SO_4)_3 \cdot 18H_2O$, is dissolved and added to the water under efficient stirring in order to ensure initial complete mixing. Aluminium hydroxide micro-flocs are produced rapidly and gathered into larger easily settling flocs. Thereafter the mixture is allowed to settle. During this flocculation process many kinds of micro-particles and negatively charged ions including fluoride are partially removed by electrostatic attachment to the flocs (equations 7–10):

Alum dissolution:
$$Al_2 (SO_4)_3 \cdot 18H_2O = 2Al^{3+} + 3SO_4^{2-} + 18H_2O \qquad (7)$$

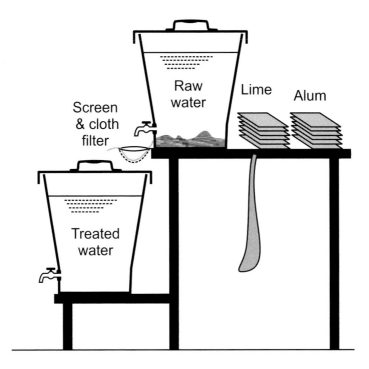

Figure 5.6   The Nalgonda defluoridation as adopted for domestic use in the United Republic of Tanzania. After Dahi *et al.*, 1996.

Aluminium precipitation (Acidic):
$$2Al^{3+} + 6H_2O = 2Al(OH)_3 + 6H^+ \tag{8}$$

Co-precipitation *(non*-stoichiometric, undefined product):
$$F^- + Al(OH)_3 = Al–F \text{ complex} + \text{undefined product} \tag{9}$$

pH adjustment:
$$6Ca(OH)_2 + 12H^+ = 6Ca^{2+} + 12H_2O \tag{10}$$

Compared with normal drinking-water flocculation, a much larger dosage of aluminium sulfate is normally required in the defluoridation process. As the aluminium sulfate solution is acidic, simultaneous addition of lime is often needed to ensure neutral pH in the treated water and complete precipitation of aluminium. Surplus lime is used as a weighting agent, i.e. to facilitate more complete settling. The treated water can be decanted. Filtration is, however,

required as a polishing stage in order to ensure that no sludge particles escape
with the treated water.

5.4.2 Technical configuration

The Nalgonda defluoridation techniques was developed for African households
as shown in Figure 5.6. Aluminium sulfate and lime are sold to the consumers as
powders in small sealed differently marked plastic bags. One set of two bags
contains the dosages required to defluoridate one bucket of water. The treatment
system consists of two locally available 20 litre plastic buckets, each supplied
with one small brass tap of the type used for domestic filter containers. The taps
are fixed 5 cm above the bottom of the buckets in order to enable trapping of
sludge below the draw-off point. The upper bucket tap is fitted with a tea sieve on
which a piece of cotton cloth is placed, allowing the water to flow directly into
the second clean water bucket.

   Aluminium sulfate and lime are added simultaneously to the raw water
bucket where they are dissolved/suspended by stirring with a wooden paddle.
The villagers are trained to stir fast while counting to 60 (1 minute) and then
slowly while counting to 300 (5 minutes). The flocs formed are left to settle for
about one hour. The treated water is then run from the tap through the cloth into
the treated water bucket from where it is stored for daily drinking and cooking.

   It has been shown (Dahi *et al.*, 1997) that the fluoride is only loosely bound to
the aluminium hydroxide flocs. That is why the treated water must be removed
not later than a couple of hours after initiating the flocculation, and why the
precipitate should be discarded between batches.

5.4.3 Design criteria

The batch treatment described above is suitable for a daily routine, where one
bucket of water is treated for one day's water demand. If a 20 litre bucket is used,
the bucket should be filled with only 18 litres to allow for efficient mixing with
chemicals. An estimate of the amounts of alum required may be calculated using
the Freundlich based equation as developed by Dahi *et al.* (1997):

$$A = \frac{\left(F_r - F_t\right) \times V}{\alpha \times F_t^{1/\beta}}$$

Where:

A	is the amount of aluminium sulfate required, g
F_r	is the fluoride concentration in the raw water, mg l^{-1}
F_t	is the residual fluoride concentration in the treated water, mg l^{-1}
V	is the volume of water to be treated in batch, litres
α	is the sorption capacity constant ($1^{(1-1/\beta)} \times$ mg$^{2/\beta}$) g^{-1}
β	is the sorption intensity constant (dimensionless).

Any resulting pH between 6.2 and 7.6 is close to optimum. For pH = 6.7 and required residual fluoride between 1 and 1.5 mg l^{-1}, α = 6 and β = 1.33. The amount of lime required to achieve the optimum pH is difficult to estimate theoretically because it depends on the quality of lime, the alkalinity and pH of the raw water and the fluoride removal itself. According to Dahi *et al.* (1997) lime addition may be 20–50 per cent of the alum dosage.

5.4.4 Cost

According to COWI (1998) the price of one of the above buckets in the United Republic of Tanzania was about TZS 3,000 or about US$ 3.3 at 1995 prices. The tap would cost about US$ 1.7. Seven pairs of aluminium sulfate and lime bags cost US$ 0.15. Of this price, 20 per cent represents the purchase of chemicals. Aluminium sulfate is purchased on a tax-free wholesale basis, as for water works.

5.4.5 Sludge disposal

Discarding the sludge from the Nalgonda process is often thought of as a serious environmental health problem. The sludge is quite toxic because it contains the removed fluoride in a concentrated form. The sludge retained in the empty raw water bucket is to be discarded in a pit or a soakaway:

- inaccessible to children;
- inaccessible to animals;
- away from the kitchen garden; and
- remote from wells which may be used for drinking.

Once these precautions are taken, the sludge would be of low or no environmental health significance, provided only drinking and cooking water is treated. In nature the fluoride would be expected to immobilize rapidly due to weathering processes. The free fluoride ion would then be subject to infiltration or run off.

5.4.6 Experience

The aluminium sulfate and lime process was proposed for defluoridation of water when fluoride in water became a health concern in the USA as the agent behind mottling of teeth (Boruff, 1934). Four decades later the process was adopted by NEERI as the Nalgonda technique and developed for low cost use at all levels in India (Nawlakhe *et al.*, 1975). Figures 5.7 and 5.8 illustrate configurations of the Nalgonda technique at village community and water works levels. At the community level, the Nalgonda process can be linked to a single tubewell using a "draw and fill" method as shown in Figure 5.7. In larger systems (for instance where tubewells are linked to a distribution system) the Nalgonda

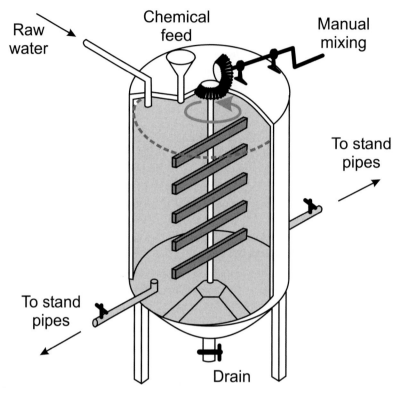

Figure 5.7   The fill and draw type Nalgonda technique for domestic and community defluoridation. After Bulusu *et al.*, 1993.

process can be incorporated into a treatment train using flash mixing before floc-culation as in Figure 5.8. The comprehensive studies on the Nalgonda technique at NEERI have resulted in three main achievements:

- The widespread knowledge about the possibilities of solving the treatment problems at different levels, even at very low cost.
- Understanding of the non-stoichiometric co-precipitation mechanisms for removal of fluoride in the flocculation process.
- The dosage design given as a simple table nomogram, indicating the required dosage of aluminium sulfate for given values of water alkalinity and fluoride concentrations. The dosage of lime is fixed at 5 per cent of the added aluminium sulfate (Bulusu *et al.*, 1993).

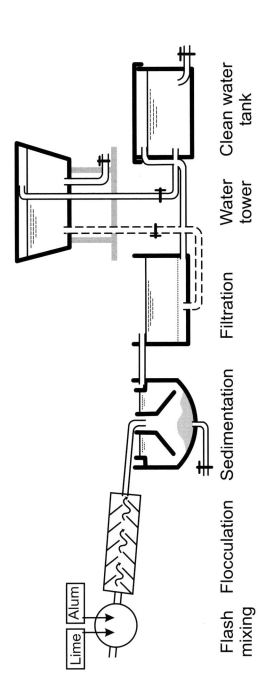

Flash mixing   Flocculation   Sedimentation   Filtration   Water tower   Clean water tank

Figure 5.8 The Nalgonda process as installed in the United Republic of Tanzania.

The mixing of the alum may be manual or using electronic paddles, depending on the size of the supply and skill of the operators. Although there are some favourable comments about the application of the Nalgonda process at community supply levels, there appears to be an increasing move towards promotion of household units in India. It has been noted by UNICEF that, although in principle community units fixed to hand pumps result in lower-costs per capita of de-fluoridation, sustainability is often problematic. Community-level water treatment of any sort is difficult to sustain because the skills required are often significant and, in the case of a process such as Nalgonda, treatment requires a significant time commitment by operators to ensure that it is effective. In community settings, ensuring such commitments may be difficult.

Household treatment options appear to offer greater potential for sustained use, in part because overall time commitments may be lower and also because the benefits to the user are more directly obvious. However, such approaches are not without problems, for instance the need for an efficient and effective service network to ensure that filters can be replaced or regenerated. UNICEF now promotes household rather than community-treatment. Although there have been references to the effectiveness of Nalgonda at a household level, there is a need for further evaluation of its effectiveness. In India there has been some move towards the use of activated alumina, although the household Nalgonda process is still promoted.

The above-mentioned design was not found to be useful for African waters of relatively high fluoride content and low alkalinity. Furthermore, for African waters it was found that lime should be added at a much higher dosage in order to achieve the pH for optimum removal. Accordingly, a more appropriate mathematical tool for the design was developed (Dahi *et al.*, 1997).

In spite of the fact that the Nalgonda technique has been introduced in many places, it has not yet been demonstrated to be the method of choice. It certainly has the great advantages of being cheap, simple and based on widely available chemicals and materials. Yet experience has shown that the following may play a role as negative factors:

- The treatment efficiency is limited to about 70 per cent. Thus the process would be less satisfactory in case of medium to high fluoride contamination in the raw water.
- A large dose of aluminium sulfate, up to 700–1,200 mg l^{-1}, may be needed. Thus it reaches the threshold where the users start complaining about residual sulfate salinity in the treated water. The large dose also results in a large sludge disposal problem in the case of water works treatment.
- When the users are not properly instructed, this can result in a large effort in terms of unnecessarily long mixing times.

It is often stated that much care has to be taken to avoid the presence of aluminium in the treated water. This is because the WHO guideline value for aluminium of 0.2 mg l^{-1} is adopted as a compromise between the technical use in drinking-water treatment and the discolouration of distributed water. Experience has demonstrated that the risk of water contamination has been highly overstated. Practically speaking it is only necessary to avoid the escape of flocs. This is easily done by careful draining of the supernatant water in combination with simple filtration as a second barrier.

5.5   Activated alumina

5.5.1 Description

Activated alumina is aluminium oxide (Al_2O_3) grains prepared to have a sorptive surface. When the water passes through a packed column of activated alumina, pollutants and other components in the water are adsorbed onto the surface of the grains (see Equation (1), section 5.1.3). Eventually the column becomes saturated: first at its upstream zone and later, as more water is passed through, the saturated zone moves downstream with the column eventually becoming totally saturated.

Total saturation means that the concentration of fluoride in the effluent water increases to the same value as the influent water. Total saturation of the column must be avoided. The column should only be operated to a *break point*, where the effluent concentration is, for example, 2 mg l^{-1} at *normal saturation*. The time between the start of operation and reaching the break point of the column is represented by V, the accumulated volume of treated water. When dividing V by the bulk volume of the packed activated alumina, a standard operational parameter is obtained; i.e. the number of Bed Volumes, BV. BV is an expression of the capacity of treatment before the column medium needs to be renewed or regenerated and is highly dependent on the raw water fluoride concentration.

5.5.2 Technical configuration

The activated alumina process is carried out in sorption filters as shown in Figure 5.3. In order to avoid the monitoring of the water quality, the unit is supplied with a water meter allowing for direct indication of the cumulative water flow. After treatment of, for example, 2,000 litres equivalent to 250 BV of water containing about 5 mg l^{-1}, the unit is opened for renewal of the 8 kg of medium. Alternatively the unit is dismounted for regeneration by the dealer.

5.5.3 *Regeneration*

Regeneration of the saturated alumina is carried out by exposing the medium to 4 per cent caustic soda (NaOH) either in batch or by flow through the column, resulting in a few BV of caustic wastewater contaminated with fluoride. Residual caustic soda is then washed out and the medium is neutralized with a 2 per cent sulfuric acid rinse.

During this process about 5–10 per cent of the alumina is lost, and the capacity of the remaining medium is reduced by 30–40 per cent. After 3–4 regenerations the medium has to be replaced. Alternatively, in order to avoid on-site regeneration, the saturated alumina can be recycled to a dealer, who can adjust the capacity of the activated alumina to the desired value by using an appropriate mixture of fresh and regenerated media.

Where the process is operated at domestic level, the regeneration cannot be left to the users. Instead, a central chemical store is set up in each village, where the users can get the regeneration done along with motivation and encouragement to continue the fluorosis prevention.

Regeneration may result in the presence of aluminium at a concentration greater than 0.2 mg l^{-1} if the pH is not readjusted to normal.

5.5.4 *Design criteria*

The alumina process is designed as a sorption process according to the same principle as bone charcoal (see Table 5.4). Similar considerations about the flow and the mix are valid. Also in the case of alumina the key design parameter is the operational defluoridation capacity, which may deviate from the theoretical capacity.

According to Hao and Huang (1986) the fluoride removal capacity of alumina is between 4 and 15 mg g^{-1}. Experience from the field, however, shows that the removal capacity is often about 1 mg g^{-1} (COWI, 1998). Thus there seems to be a large difference in the degree of "activation" of alumina products. One of the explanations may be due to variation in pH. The capacity of alumina is highly dependent on pH, the optimum being about pH 5. While it may be easy to adjust pH for maximum removal at a waterworks, it is necessary to depend on the actual pH of the raw water in domestic and small community treatments. Other explanations are the brand or source of the product. This variability demonstrates the importance of carrying out field trials. For the design the capacity of the available alumina has to be established through testing under authentic conditions. As a preliminary qualified guess, the removal capacity of 1 mg l^{-1} and the bulk density of 1.2 kg l^{-1} may be used.

Table 5.6   Some defluoridation unit prices of an NGO development project in India

Item of activated alumina	Cost (Irp)	Item of Nalgonda	Cost (Irp)
Defluoridator per unit + incl. 3 kg AA	1,200	Defluoridator per unit	500
Activated alumina per kg	65	Aluminium sulfate per kg	3
Sodium hydroxide per kg	26	Lime per kg	4
Sulphuric acid 92% per kg	8	Jerry cans, 2 pieces	160
Salary per regeneration of 3 kg	10	Measuring cylinder	60

Source: COWI (1998)

5.5.5 *Cost*

It was previously considered that the activated alumina process, due to high chemical cost and non-availability in markets, was not a consideration for most developing countries. This is no longer the case. Experience, mainly from India, Thailand and China, indicates that activated alumina may under certain conditions be affordable for low income communities. Table 5.6 compares the costs of activated alumina treatment with those of the Nalgonda process.

5.5.6 *Experience*

Activated alumina was proposed for defluoridation of water and a drum filter (see Figure 5.3) was patented for domestic use as early as 1936 (Fink and Lindsay, 1936). Since then activated alumina has become the subject of several patents and, due to commercial interests, one of the most advocated defluoridation methods.

The activated alumina process was evaluated for fluoride removal from an underground mine water in South Africa in the early 1980s and it was found that potable water could be produced from an underground mine water with a fluoride concentration of approximately 8 mg l^{-1}. Two 500×10^3 litres per day defluoridation plants were installed as a result of the investigation (Schoeman 1987a,b; Schoeman and Botha, 1985).

As the ceramic candle domestic filter is well known in some countries, it has been used as a unit for activated alumina defluoridation, although not specifically designed for it. In a special modification, the "candles" are replaced with a connection screen and a wing nut for adjustment of the filtration rate.

Activated alumina is a widely available industrial chemical. It is, however, not as widely distributed at the grass roots level as aluminium sulfate. Furthermore, its use has been limited by the difficulties of regeneration, the low capacity of less purified technical grade products and the relatively high price. Activated alumina has become less costly and more popular, especially where it is manufactured.

5.6   Clay

5.6.1 Description

Clay is an earthy sedimentary material composed mainly of fine particles of hydrous aluminium silicates and other minerals and impurities. Clay is fine-textured, plastic when moist, retains its shape when dried and sinters hard when fired. These properties are utilized in manufacture of pottery, brick and tile. Both clay powder and fired clay are capable of sorption of fluoride as well as other pollutants from water. The ability of clay to clarify turbid water is well known. This property is believed to have been known and utilized at domestic level in ancient Egypt.

5.6.2 Technical configuration

Although clay takes up fluoride as in a sorption process, it may be used as a flocculent powder in a batch system like the one shown in Figure 5.6. Because clay has a relatively high density, e.g. compared to bone charcoal, it will settle and enable decanting or drain off of the supernatant water. The use of clay powder in columns is possible, but troublesome mainly because of difficulties in packing the columns and controlling the flow.

Domestic clay column filters are therefore normally packed using clay chips found as waste from the manufacture of brick, pottery or tile. Figure 5.9 illustrates such a column filter. It resembles the filter used in Sri Lanka and reported by Padmasiri (1998). The filter is based on up-flow in order to allow for settling of suspended solids within the filter bed. The filter does not have a clean water reservoir and the filtration rate is controlled by slow withdrawal through the tap.

The column described by Padmasiri (1998) is stratified with one layer of charred coconut shells and another layer of pebbles above the entire bed of brick chips. Depending on the raw water quality, and on the quality of the brick chips, such a post-filtration through charcoal may be a precondition to obtain good water quality. As charcoal has a low specific density, the pebbles stabilize the stratified bed and are necessary to avoid the escape of charcoal grains with the treated water.

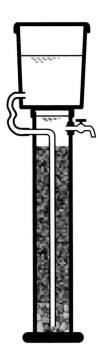

Figure 5.9   Stratified column of brick chips, pebbles and coconut shells as used in Sri Lanka.

5.6.3 Regeneration

Clay and similar media can be regenerated, at least partially. It would not, however, be cost effective in most cases.

5.6.4 Design criteria

Based on testing of the capacity of clay to remove fluoride from water, different studies reach different conclusions about the capacity and usability of the method in general. Thus, Zevenbergen *et al.* (1996) conclude that "*the Ando soil appears to be an economical and efficient method for defluoridation of drinking water*" while Bulusu *et al.* (1979) do not find the clay worth mentioning as a defluoridation agent.

According to the study of Zevenbergen *et al.* (1996) the defluoridation capacity of the Ando soil of Kenya was 5.5 mg g^{-1} while Moges *et al.* (1996) found that the capacity of ground and fired clay pot of Ethiopia was no more than 0.2 mg g^{-1}. It could be concluded that the Ando soil of Kenya was more efficient in defluoridating the water than the clay pot powder of Ethiopia. Examination of the data indicated that this was not the case. If the use of the Ando soil studied by Zevenbergen *et al.* (1996) was simulated under authentic field conditions in a bucket treatment system, it revealed defluoridation capacity of the same order as studied by Moges *et al.* (1996), i.e. about 0.2 mg g^{-1}.

Bårdsen and Björvatn (1997) studied the sorption isotherm of clay calcined at 600 °C. They found that the sorption continues to take place even up to 10 days of contact time, but the capacity was as low as 0.07 mg g^{-1} at 1 mg l^{-1} level. Thus in order to remove 3.4 mg l^{-1} of fluoride from water containing fluoride at a level as high as 12.5 mg l^{-1}, within one hour of contact time, they had to add calcined clay at a level of 100 g l^{-1}, i.e. batch operational capacity of 0.03 mg g^{-1}. Convincing field experiments have been reported by Padmasiri (1998) showing an operational capacity of 0.08 mg g^{-1} for brick chips used in column defluoridators in Sri Lanka. According to Jinadasa *et al.* (1988), the capacity is known to be optimum when pH is about 5.6.

For design purposes the operational capacity has to be investigated first. As a preliminary guideline the capacities of 0.03 and 0.1 mg g^{-1} may be used respectively for design of batch and column defluoridators using clay materials, as shown in Table 5.7 for example. Because the clay powder in a bucket system is to be added at large dosages, the volume of the treated water wasted along with the sludge has to be considered. From the design examples shown in Table 5.7 it may be seen that the dosages required are estimated to be 73 and 20 g l^{-1} respectively. Thus the dosage is much higher than in the other methods, even though the raw water fluoride is as low as 3 mg l^{-1}. Furthermore, the removal efficiencies are expected to be low, i.e. 67 per cent. Probably the clay process would be of no, or at least much less, use if the water contains higher concentrations of fluoride or if better removal efficiencies are required.

5.6.5 Hygienic precautions

Clay and most other soil minerals which demonstrate defluoridation capacities are primarily cation-exchangers. Toxic heavy metals and a wide range of other pollutants may also be retained in the clay strata when rain water percolates soil. Care has therefore to be taken in order to ensure that for any soil material to be used in a defluoridation process:

- the medium should be calcined and stored hygienically;
- the medium loses its defluoridation capacity if calcined to dead burnt temperatures, e.g. 1,200 °C;
- the medium should be tested for potential dissolution of toxic materials; and
- the medium should not support for microbial growth due to the content of organic carbon.

5.6.6 Cost

It has been stated by Padmasiri (1998) that the clay process is only cost effective if the freshly burnt broken bricks of good quality are available on site or adjacent to the users and if the filter is prepared using low cost, locally available materials.

5.6.7 Experience

According to Padmasiri (1998) nearly 80 per cent of 600 clay column defluoridators installed in households in Sri Lanka were found in operating condition after being monitored for different periods from two years onwards. The described technology was found to be sustainable, but only if the users were motivated through information and motivation campaigns (COWI, 1998).

5.7 Evaluation and selection of method

The above reporting on the methods of defluoridation reveals that there is not a universal method which is appropriate under all social, financial, economic, environmental and technical conditions. None of the methods has been implemented successfully at a large scale in many parts of the world. This is quite remarkable, especially when taking into consideration the fact that several defluoridation methods have been studied in detail and even reported as appropriate methods, for a number of years (Bulusu *et al.*, 1979). Apart from contact precipitation, all the methods were known as early as the mid-1930s when the agent behind "the Colorado stain" was discovered. This oddity is probably because all available defluoridation methods do have disadvantages. Some of these are what may be designated as killer disadvantages, in the sense that the methods turn out to be unsustainable under the given socio-economical conditions. Such killer disadvantages of defluoridation or of some defluoridation techniques in particular circumstances include:

1. *High Cost-Tech;* i.e. either the price and/or the technology is high, demanding imported spare parts, continuous power supply, expensive chemicals, skilled operation or regeneration, etc. Reverse osmosis, ion exchange and activated alumina may thus be categorized as high cost-tech methods.
2. *Limited efficiency;* i.e. the method does not permit sufficient removal of the fluoride, even when appropriate dosage is used. As in the Nalgonda technique, the residual concentration would often be higher than 1 mg l^{-1}, unless the raw water concentration itself is relatively low as discussed above in relation to the United Republic of Tanzania.
3. *Unobserved break through;* i.e. the fluoride concentration in the treated water may rise gradually or suddenly, typically when a medium in a treatment column is exhausted or even when the flow is out of control. As in the

Table 5.7 Examples of design of bucket flocculation as illustrated in Figure 5.3 and an up flow column filter.

Parameters		Unit	Design examples	
			Bucket type	Column type
Given:				
D	Daily personal water demand	l/(c × d)	3	3
N	Number of users	p	6	6
OP	Operation period	days	1	180
Γ_o	Operational sorption capacity	g kg^{-1}	0.03	0.1
σ	Bulk density of medium (powder and chips)	kg l^{-1}	1.05	0.86
F_i	Raw water fluoride concentration	mg l^{-1}	3	3
F_t	Treated water average fluoride concentration	mg l^{-1}	1	1
$VR_{SW/M}$	Volume ratio supernatant water/medium	–	–	1/5
$VR_{AF/M}$	Volume ratio after-filter water/medium	–	–	½
$VR_{S/Q}$	Volume ratio of sludge/water demand	–	1/10	–
$VR_{VS/Q}$	Volume ratio vacant space for mix/water demand	–	1/15	–

Continued

Table 5.7   Continued.

Parameters		Unit	Design examples	
			Bucket type	Column type
Derived:				
$Q = D \times N$	Daily water treatment	l/d	18	18
$V_S = Q \times VR_{S/Q}$	Volume of residual sludge	l	2	–
$V_T = OP \times Q + V_S$	Total volume of water treated in a filter period	l	20	3,200
$F_T = V_T \times (F_i - F_t)\,/\,1{,}000$	Total fluoride removal during a period	g	0.04	6
$M = F_T / \Gamma_o$	Amount of medium required for renewal	kg	1.3	65
$V_M = M / \sigma$	Volume of medium in the filter	l	0.9	50
$BV = V_T / V_M$	Number of bed volumes treated in a filter period	–	–	45
$V_{SW} = V_M \times VR_{SW/M}$	Volume capacity of supernatant water	l	–	15
$V_{AF} = V_M / V_{AF/M}$	Volume of after-filter arrangement	l	–	40
$V_{VS} = Q \times VR_{VS/Q}$	Volume capacity of vacant space in bucket	l	1.2	0
$V_B = Q + V_S + V_{VS}$; $V_F = V_M + V_{SW} + V_{AF}$	Total volume of bucket/filter	l	40	130
Corresponding dimensions:				
Ø	Filter diameter (selected as available)	cm	35	40
$H = V_B / (\pi \times (\text{Ø}/2)^2)$ or $V_F / (\pi \times (\text{Ø}/2)^2)$	Total height of the bucket/filter	cm	40	100

It is assumed that clay powder having capacity 0.03 mg g^{-1} and bulk density of 1.5 kg g^{-1} in the bucket type filter. The column filter utilizes clay brick grains of 8–16 mm, the capacity being 0.1 mg g^{-1} and the bulk density 1.3 kg l^{-1}.

Table 5.8   General comparison of advantages of the most promising
defluoridation methods.

Advantages	Defluoridation method				
	BC	CP	NaI	AA	Cl
No daily dosage of chemicals, i.e. no daily working load	+	–	–	+	+
Dosage designed for actual F conc. independent of unit or plant	–	+	+	–	–
No risk of false treatment due to break point	–	+	+	–	–
Removal capacity of medium is independent of F concentration	–	+	–	–	–
No regeneration or renewal of medium is required	–	+	+	–	–
High removal efficiency can be ensured	+	+	–	+	–
Easy to construct, even by the users	+	+	++	+	+
Construction materials are cheap and widely available	+	+	++	+	+
Can be sized for one or several families or a group, e.g. a school	+	++	+	+	–
No risk of medium/chemicals unacceptability	–	–/+	+	+	–
No risk of deterioration of the original water quality	–/+	+	–/+	–/+	–

BC = bone charcoal; CP = contact precipitation; NaI = Nalgonda technique of aluminium
sulfate and lime; AA = activated alumina; Cl = calcined clay
"risk" means in some cases
+ indicates advantage; – indicates potential disadvantage

case of bone charcoal and other column filters, these techniques necessitate frequent monitoring of fluoride residual, or at least the rate and the volume of treated water, if unobserved breakthrough or the loss of removal capacity are to be avoided.

4. *Limited capacity;* while the removal capacity of bone charcoal or activated alumina may be about 2 mg of fluoride per gram of medium, much higher amounts of calcined clay for example have to be used in order to obtain appropriate removal.

5. *Deteriorated water quality;* this would by nature result in excessively high pH values, normally above 10. The water quality may also deteriorate due to poorly prepared medium (bone charcoal) or due to medium escaping from the treatment container, e.g. ion exchange, alumina, Nalgonda sludge, etc.

6. *Taboo limitations;* in particular, the bone charcoal method is culturally not acceptable to Hindus. Bone charcoal originating from pigs may be questioned by Muslims. The charring of bones has also been reported to be unacceptable to villagers in North Thailand.

By contrast, all the methods mentioned do have advantages and have been shown to be capable of removing fluoride under certain conditions. Four criteria are essential and may contribute to the success of fluorosis prevention through treatment of drinking-water at a decentralized level:

1. The right method has to be selected to deal with given water quality and social acceptability. Table 5.8 may be useful in selection of the method.
2. Proper design and process understanding are required at least among the responsible officials.
3. Media and unit spare parts have to be made available though an appropriate infrastructure, such as village communities and social and health workers.
4. Motivation and training of users has to be continued through the same, or a similar, infrastructure.

Research and development and experience in this field continues to develop and care must be taken to seek further information, whether the requirement is for small scale treatment using cheap, locally available, materials, or for larger scale systems.

5.8 References

AWWA 1971 Defluoridation of water. In: *Water Quality and Treatment.* 3rd Edition, McGraw-Hill, 436–440.

Bårdsen, A. and Björvatn, K. 1997 Fluoride sorption in fired clay. In: *Proceedings of the First International Workshop on Fluorosis and Defluoridation of Water*, 18–22 October 1995, Tanzania, The International Society for Fluoride Research, Auckland, 46–49.

Björvatn, K. and Bårdsen, A. 1997 Use of activated clay for defluoridation of water. In: *Proceedings of the First International Workshop on Fluorosis and Defluoridation of Water*, 18–22 October 1995, Tanzania, The International Society for Fluoride Research, Auckland, 40–45.

Boruff, C.S. 1934 Removal of fluorides from drinking waters. *Industrial and Engineering Chemistry,* **25** (Jan), 69–71.

Bower, C.A. and Hatcher, J.T. 1967 Adsorption of fluoride by soils and minerals. *Soil Science*, **103** (3), 151–154.

Bregnhøj, H., Dahi, E. and Jensen, M. 1997 Modelling defluoridation of water in bone char columns. In: *Proceedings of the First International Workshop on Fluorosis and Defluoridation of Water*. 18–22 October 1995, Tanzania, The International Society for Fluoride Research, Auckland, 72–83.

Bulusu, K.R., Nawlakhe, W.G., Patil, A.R. and Karthikeyan, G. 1993 *Water Quality and Defluoridation Techniques.* Volume 11 of Prevention and Control of Fluorosis, Rajiv Gandhi National Drinking Water Mission, Ministry of Rural Development, New Delhi.

Bulusu, K.R., Sundaresan, B.B., Pathak, B.N., Nawlakhe, W.G. *et al.*, 1979 Fluorides in water, defluoridation methods and their limitations. *Journal of the Institution of Engineers (India,* **60,** 1–25.

COWI 1998 *Review of Practical experiences with defluoridation in rural water supply programmes Part 11.* Ministry of Foreign Affairs, Danida, Copenhagen, 73 pp.

Dahi, E. 1996 Contact precipitation for defluoridation of water. Paper presented at 22nd WEDC Conference, New Delhi, 9–13 September 1996.

Dahi, E. 1998 Small community plants for low cost defluoridation of water by contact precipitation. In: *Proceedings of the 2nd International Workshop on Fluorosis and Defluoridation of Water.* Nazareth, 19–22 November 1997, The International Society for Fluoride Research, Auckland.

Dahi, E. and Bregnhøj, H. 1997 Significance of oxygen in processing of bone char for defluoridation of water. In: *Proceedings of the First International Workshop on Fluorosis and Defluoridation of Water,* 18–22 October 1995, Tanzania, The International Society for Fluoride Research, Auckland, 84–90.

Dahi, E., Bregnhøj, H. and Orio, L. 1997 Sorption isotherms of fluoride on flocculated alumina. In: *Proceedings of the First International Workshop on Fluorosis and Defluoridation of Water.* 18–22 October 1995, Tanzania, The International Society for Fluoride Research, Auckland, 35–39.

Dahi, E., Mtalo, F., Njau, B. and Bregnhøj, H. 1996 Defluoridation using the Nalgonda Technique in Tanzania. Paper presented at the 22nd WEDC Conference, India, New Delhi, 1996.

Dunckley, G.G. and Malthus, R.S. 1961 Removal of fluoride from fluoridated water. *New Zealand Journal of Science,* **4,** 504.

Fink, G.J. and Lindsay, F.K. 1936 Activated alumina for removing fluorides from drinking water. *Industrial and Engineering,* **28** (9), 947–948.

Hao, O.J. and Huang, C.P. 1986 Adsorption characteristics of fluoride onto hydrous alumina. *Journal of Environmental Engineering,* **112** (6), 1054–1069.

Heidweiller, V.M.L. 1992 Fluoride removal methods. In: Frencken, J.E. (Ed.) *Endemic Fluorosis In Developing Countries: Causes, Effects and Possible Solutions*, Report of a Symposium held in Delft, the Netherlands, NIPG-TNO, Leiden.

Jacobsen, P. and Dahi, E. 1998 Low cost domestic defluoridation of drinking water by means of locally charred bone. In: *Proceedings of the 2nd International Workshop on Fluorosis and Defluoridation of Water.* Nazareth, 19–22 November 1997, The International Society for Fluoride Research, Auckland.

Jinadasa, K.B.P.N., Weerasooriya, S.W.R. and Dissanayake, C.B. 1988 A rapid method for the defluoridation of fluoride-rich drinking waters at village level. *International Journal of Environmental Studies,* **31,** 305–312.

Mantell, C.L. 1968 Bone char. *Carbone and Graphite Handbook.* Interscience Publishers, New York, 538 pp, SBN 470 56779.

Maruthamuthu, M. and Venkatanarayana, R. 1987 A native index of defluoridation by serpentine. *Fluoride,* **20** (2), 64–67.

Moges, G., Zwenge, F. and Socher, M. 1996 Preliminary investigations on the defluoridation of water using fired clay chips. *Journal of African Earth Science,* **21** (4), 479–482.

Nawlakhe, W.G., Kulkarni, D.N., Pathak, B.N. and Bulusu, K.R. 1975 Defluoridation of water by Nalgonda Technique. *Indian Journal of Environmental Health,* **17** (1), 26–65.

Padmasiri, J.P. 1998 Low cost defluoridation of drinking water by means of brick chips. In: *Proceedings of the 2nd International Workshop on Fluorosis and Defluoridation of Water.* Nazareth, 19–22 November 1997, The International Society for Fluoride Research, Auckland.

Padmasiri, J.P. and Dissanayake, C.B. 1995 A simple defluoridator for removing excess fluorides from fluoride-rich drinking water. *International Journal of Environmental Health Research,* **5,** 153–160.

Phantumvanit, P., Songpaisan, Y. and Møller, I.J. 1988 A defluoridator for individual households. *World Health Forum.* **9** (4), 555–558.

Roche, E.H. 1968 A fluoride filter for domestic use. *New Zealand Dental Journal.* **64,** 18–22.

Schoeman, J. J. and Botha, G. R. 1985 An evaluation of the activated alumina process for fluoride removal from drinking water and some factors influencing its performance. *Water SA,* **11** (1), 25–32.

Schoeman, J. J. 1987a An investigation of the performance of two newly installed defluoridation plants in South Africa and some factors affecting its performance. *Water Science and Technology,* **19**, 953–965.

Schoeman, J. J. 1987b The effect of particle size and interfering ions on fluoride removal by activated alumina. *Water SA,* **13** (4), 229–234.

Singano, J.J., Mashauri, D.A., Dahi, E. and Mtalo, F.W. 1997 Effect of pH on defluoridation of water by magnesite. *Proceedings of the First International Workshop on Fluorosis and Defluoridation of Water.* 18–22 October 1995, Tanzania, The International Society for Fluoride Research, Auckland, 30–34.

Zevenbergen, C., van Reeuvijk, L.P., Louws, R.J. and Schuiling, R.D. 1996 A simple method for defluoridation of drinking water at village level by adsorption on ando soil in Kenya. *The Science of the Total Environment,* **188,** 225–232.

6

Analytical methods

This chapter gives an overview of the most commonly used primary analytical methods for laboratory determination of total fluoride in drinking-water. Sample handling and pre-treatment are covered, on a matrix basis. Several methods are described in the literature for the analysis of total fluoride, both in water and in different digested matrices. Preference is given here to widely used international or national standard methods, which are prescribed for use in many laboratories and which have been validated prior to issue. Rapid field test kits, ion-selective electrode (pH meter) method and Complexone method 2 (Nova 60 instrument made by Merck Co.) are also explained. The possible analytical methods for fluoride determination include:

- Ion-chromatography (IC): *laboratory test*
  - Chemical Suppression of Eluent Conductivity Method (EPA 300.0, ASTM D4327-91 and Standard Methods 4110B, ISO 10359-1)
- Ion-selective electrode (pH meter): *field and laboratory test*
  - Ion-selective Electrode Method (ASTM D1179-93B and Standard Methods 4500F-C)
- Colorimetry
  - Complexone Method 1 (EPA 340.3, Standard Methods 4500F-E): *laboratory test*
  - Complexone Method 2 (EPA 340.3, Standard Methods 4500F-E): *field and laboratory test*
  - SPANDNS Method (Standard Methods 4500F-D): *laboratory test*

To achieve a sufficiently low detection limit using any of the techniques all of the reagents must be free of fluoride. The quality of the reagents needs to be carefully selected and evaluated to maintain the blank as low as possible. All the techniques require trained staff, generally analysts experienced in dealing with trace elements, with facilities to deal with potentially hazardous chemicals. In addition to any specialized equipment specified for the analysis, all the techniques require the use of standard laboratory equipment.

6.1 Ion-chromatography with chemical suppression of eluent conductivity

Determination of the fluoride anion is necessary for the characterization of water and/or to assess the need for specific treatment and to determine the efficacy of treatment. This technique of Ion Chromatography (IC) uses non-hazardous reagents and it effectively distinguishes between halides and oxy-anions. This method is applicable, after filtration to remove particles larger than 0.2 μm, to surface waters, groundwaters, wastewaters, and drinking-water.

The standard conditions of IC when using the Dionex DX500 ion chromatograph are:

Ion Chromatograph:	Dionex DX500
Columns:	Dionex AG9-HC/AS9-HC, 2 mm
Detector:	Suppressed Conductivity Detector, Dionex CD20
Suppressor:	ASRS-I, external source electrolyte mode, 100 mA current
Eluent:	9.0 mM Na_2CO_3
Eluent flow:	0.40 ml per minute
Sample loop:	10 μl
System backpressure:	2,800 psi
Background conductivity:	22 μS

Method and performance characteristics
A small volume of sample is introduced into an ion chromatograph as shown in Figure 6.1. The anions are separated on the basis of their relative affinities for a low capacity, strongly basic anion exchanger (guard and separator columns). The separated anions, in their acid forms after the suppressor, are measured by conductivity. They are identified on the basis of retention time as compared to standards (SM4110: 1999). Reproducibility, expressed as relative standard deviations, is found in reagent tests (0.26–8.49 mg l^{-1}) to be 0–15 per cent.

Interference and matrix effects
Interferences can be divided into three different categories: 1) direct chromatographic co-elution, in which an analyte response is observed at very nearly the

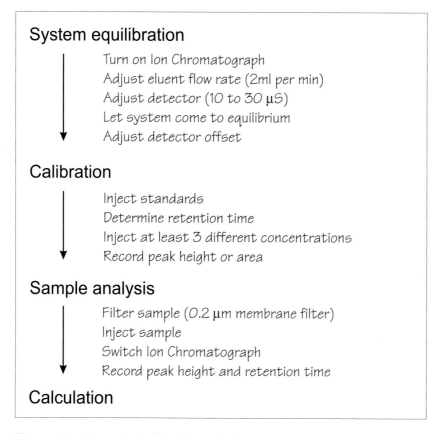

Figure 6.1   Flow chart of fluoride analysis by ion chromatography.

same retention time as the target anion; 2) concentration dependent co-elution, which is observed when the response to higher than typical concentrations of a neighbouring peak overlap into the retention window of the target anion; and 3) ionic character displacement, where retention times may shift significantly due to the influence of high ionic strength matrices (high mineral content or hardness) overloading the exchange sites in the column and significantly shortening the analyte's retention times.

A direct chromatographic co-elution may be solved by changing columns, eluent strength, modifying the eluent with organic solvents, changing the detection systems, or selective removal of the interference with pre-treatment. Sample dilution may resolve some of the difficulties if the interference is the result of either concentration dependent or ionic character displacement. Pre-treatment cartridges can be effective for eliminating certain matrix interferences.

Usually, fluoride is difficult to quantify at low concentrations because the water that is eluted first produces a negative peak on the chromatogram, sometimes know as the "water dip", which cancels the positive peak arising from low concentrations of fluoride. Simple organic acids (formic, carbonic, etc.) elute close to fluoride and also cause interference. Fluoride can be determined accurately by using special dilute eluent or gradient elution using NaOH eluent (Clesceri *et al.*, 1998).

Sample size
Normally a sample volume of at least 1 ml is injected for a 0.1 ml sample loop; however, it is essential that the sample is representative.

Equipment and consumable requirements
An ion chromatograph equipped with an injection valve, sample loop, guard column, anion separator column, and fibre or membrane suppressors, a temperature-compensated small-volume conductivity cell and detector, and a strip-chart recorder are required. An ion chromatograph capable of delivering 2 to 5 ml eluent per minute at a pressure of 1,400–6,900 kPa should be used. The price for an ion chromatograph system is approximately US$ 30,000–60,000. Chemical consumption, which represents the main running cost, is low.

Throughput
Sample preparation is minimal, the time consuming step being the start up of the equipment. When using an auto-sampler the daily throughput for the equipment is in the range 50–70 samples a day.

Sample collection, preservation and storage
The samples should be collected in plastic or glass bottles. All bottles must be thoroughly cleaned and rinsed with reagent water. The samples collected should be representative and the volumes collected should be sufficient for replicate analysis. Sample preservation is not required but it is recommended to keep the samples cool and to analyse them within 28 days.

6.2 Ion-selective electrode method

Fluoride is determined potentiometrically using a fluoride electrode in conjunction with a standard single-junction, sleeve-type reference electrode and a pH meter having an expanded millivolt scale or a selective ion meter having a direct concentration scale for fluoride. Fluoride ion activity depends on the solution total ionic strength and pH, and on fluoride complex species. Adding an appropriate buffer provides a nearly uniform ionic strength background, adjusts the pH, and breaks up complexes so that the electrode measures concentration

Instrument calibration

↓ *Calibrate instrument to zero*

Preparation of fluoride standards

↓ *Prepare a series of standards*

Treatment of standards and samples

↓ *Prepare standard and samples (10 to 25 ml)*
Add equal volume of buffer

Measurement with electrode

↓ *Immerse electrodes in standard solutions*
Measure developed potentials while stirring
Let electrodes remain in solution for 3 minutes
Repeat measurement with samples

Calculation

Figure 6.2   Flow chart of fluoride analysis by ion-selective electrode method.

(ASTM D1179:1996, SM 4500F-C:1995, ISO 10359-1 1992). The fluoride electrode consists of a lanthanum fluoride crystal across which a potential is developed by fluoride ions. The cell may be represented by Ag/AgCl-(0.3), F-(0.001) LaF3 | test solution | reference electrode.

Method performance
In general, the quantitation range of fluoride by this method is 0.1–100 mg l^{-1}. Reproducibility, expressed as relative standard deviation, is found in proficiency tests to be 3.6–4.8 per cent with a range of synthetic samples of concentration 0.750–0.900 mg l^{-1} F. The flow chart for this method is shown in Figure 6.2.

Interference and matrix effects
Extremes of pH interfere; the sample pH should be between 5 and 9. Fluoride forms complexes with several polyvalent cations such as Si^{4+}, Fe^{3+} and Al^{3+}. The degree of interference depends on the concentration of complexing cations, the

Table 6.1 Interfering ions with Complexone Method 1

Ion	Allowable conc. (mg l^{-1})	Ion	Allowable conc. (mg l^{-1})
Al^{3+}	0.04	Cl^-	6,800
Ca^{2+}	330	Br^-	100
Co^{2+}	0.4	I^-	0.08
Cu^{2+}	0.4	NO_3^-	0.4
Fe^{3+}	0.3	NO_2^-	0.4
Mg^{2+}	<500	SO_4^{2-}	1,000
Ni^{2+}	<0.4	PO_4^-	0.4
Zn^{2+}	0.4	BO_3^{3-}	200

concentration of fluoride and complex species. The addition of pH 5.0 buffer containing a strong chelating agent preferentially complexes aluminium (the most common interference), silicon and iron, and eliminates the pH problem.

Sample size
Normally a minimum sample volume of 50 ml is needed for the analysis. It is essential that the sample is representative.

Equipment and consumables requirements
An expanded-scale or digital pH meter or ion-selective meter equipped with sleeve type reference electrode and fluoride electrode is required. In addition, a magnetic stirrer with a PTFE-coated stirring bar and timer are needed. Chemical consumption, which represents the main running cost, is low.

Throughput
Sample preparation is minimal but the time consuming step of the analysis is the start up of the equipment. When using the manual method the throughput for the equipment is in the range of 10 samples in 40 minutes.

Sample collection, preservation and storage
The samples should be collected in plastic or glass bottles. All bottles must be thoroughly cleaned and rinsed with reagent water. The samples collected should be representative and the volumes collected should be sufficient for replicate analysis. Sample preservation is not required but it is recommended that samples are kept cool.

Set-up manifold

Warm up for 30 minutes
Run a baseline with all reagents
Feed distilled water through sample line
Adjust colorimeter to obtain stable baseline

Measurement

Set sample timing at 2.5 minutes
Arrange fluoride standards in sampler
Switch sample line from distilled water to sampler
Begin analysis

Calculation

Figure 6.3   Flow chart of fluoride analysis by complexone method (automated).

6.3   Complexone method 1 (laboratory test)

The sample is distilled, either automatically or manually. The distillate is reacted with alizarin fluorine blue-lanthanum reagent. Fluoride ion reacts with the red chelate formed between lanthanum and alizarin fluorine blue at a pH of 4.5. The absorbance of the resulting blue ternary complex is measured at 620 nm. The reaction is carried out in 16 per cent v/v acetone medium, which stabilizes the colour and can increase sensitivity. If the concentration of interfering ions is below the allowable concentrations given in Table 6.1, the distillation stage can be omitted.

Method performance

The automated method is applicable to potable, surface and saline waters as well as domestic and industrial wastewaters. The range of the manual and automated methods, which can be modified by using an adjustable colorimeter, is 0.05–2.0 mg l^{-1} F. Reproducibility, expressed as relative standard deviation, is found in proficiency tests to be 3–10 per cent (SM 4500F-E). The flow charts for this method are shown in Figures 6.3 and 6.4.

Pre-treatment of sample
↓   *Distillation of samples in the distillation set*

Preparation of fluoride standards
↓   *Prepare a series of standards*

Treatment of standards and samples
↓   *Prepare standard and distillate*
         Add alizarin complexone, H_2SO_4, HNO_3 and acetone
         Wait 60 minutes

Measure at 620 nm
↓

Calculation

Figure 6.4   Flow chart of fluoride analysis by complexone method (manual).

Interferences and matrix effects

The method is free from most anionic and cationic interferences, except for aluminum, which forms an extremely stable fluoro complex, AlF_6^{3-}. This is overcome by treatment with 8-hydroxyquinoline to complex the aluminium and by subsequent extraction with chloroform. At aluminium levels below 0.2 mg l^{-1}, the extraction procedure is not required. However, normally, interferences are removed by distillation.

Sample size

Normally a minimum sample volume of 200 ml is needed for pre-treatment by distillation in the manual system. The samples collected should be representative and the volumes collected should be sufficient for replicate analysis. Sample preservation is not required but it is recommended to keep the samples cool and to analyse them within 28 days.

Equipment and consumable requirements

A fluoride manifold (continuous-flow auto-analyser system) equipped with proportioning pump, continuous filter, colorimeter and recorder is required. The

Set-up manifold

Filter turbid samples
Adjust pH within the range 5 – 8

Treatment of standards and samples

Add pre-treated samples (5 ml) into reaction cell
Close the cell and mix
Add reagent (1 dose), close the cell and shake
Leave for 2 minutes (reaction time)

Read concentration at 620 nm

Figure 6.5   Flow chart of fluoride analysis by complexone method at the range 0.1–1.5 mg l^{-1} F

price of the auto analyser unit is approximately US\$ 20,000–40,000. Chemical consumption, which represents the main running cost, is low.

Throughput
When using an automated system, the throughput is about 12 samples an hour.

Sample collection, preservation and storage
Sample preparation is minimal and the time consuming step of analysis is the start up of the equipment.

6.4   Complexone method 2 (field test)

Method performance
In a buffered, weakly acidic solution, fluoride ions react with alizarin complexone and lanthanum (III) to form a blue complex that is determined photometrically. The method is analogous to EPA 340.3 and Standard Methods 4500-F-E. This method is applicable to surface and mineral waters as well as wastewaters. The ranges of this method are 0.1–1.5 mg l^{-1} F and 1.0–20 mg l^{-1} F. Reproducibility, expressed as the coefficient of variation of the procedure, is found in proficiency tests to be ±2.2 per cent (ISO 1990). The flow chart for this method is shown in Figures 6.5 and 6.6.

Set-up manifold

| Filter turbid samples
↓ Adjust pH within the range 3 – 8

Treatment of standards and samples

Add reagent (2 ml)
Add distilled water (5 ml) and mix
Add pre-treated sample (0.5 ml) and mix
Add reagent (0.5 ml) and mix
Leave for 5 minutes (reaction time)
↓ Introduce the measurement samples into 10 mm cell

Read concentration at 620 nm

Figure 6.6   Flow chart of fluoride analysis by complexone method at the range 1–20 mg l^{-1} F.

Interference and matrix effects

Table 6.2 shows the interferences checked in solutions containing 1 and 0 mg l^{-1} F⁻ and Table 6.3 shows interferences checked in solutions containing 10 and 0 mg l^{-1} F⁻. The concentrations of foreign substances given in the tables lie below the limit at which interference occurs.

Sample size

Normally a minimum sample volume of 200 ml is needed for pre-treatment. The samples collected should be representative and the volumes collected should be sufficient for replicate analysis. Sample preservation is not required but it is recommended to keep the samples cool and to analyse them within 28 days.

Equipment and consumable requirements

Fluoride manifold equipped with recharge battery and round cell, colorimeter. The price of this analyser unit is approximately US$ 4,000–7,000. Chemical consumption, which represents the main running cost, is low.

Throughput

Sample preparation is minimal, the time consuming step of analysis being the start up of the equipment. When using this system, the throughput for the equipment is in the range 10 samples in 15 minutes.

Table 6.2 Interfering ions when detecting fluoride at the range 0.1–1.5 mg l^{-1} F (mg l^{-1} or %)

Ion	Interfering conc.	Ion	Interfering conc.
Al^{3+}	1	EDTA	0.1
Ca^{2+}	1,000	S^{2-}	10
Co^{2+}	1,000	Cl^-	10%
Cu^{2+}	10	NO_3^-	10%
Fe^{3+}	100	NO_2^-	1,000
Mg^{2+}	1,000	SO_4^{2-}	10%
Zn^{2+}	10	PO_4^{3-}	1,000

Table 6.3 Interfering ions when detecting fluoride in the range 1–20 mg l^{-1} F (mg l^{-1} or %)

Ion	Interfering conc.	Ion	Interfering conc.
Al^{3+}	5	Zn^{2+}	25
Cr^{3+}	50	EDTA	1
Cu^{2+}	25	Cl^-	20%
Ni^{2+}	10	NO_3^-	20%
Pb^{2+}	10	SO_4^{2-}	20%

6.5 SPADNS method

In the SPADNS (sodium 2-(parasulfophenylazo)–1,8–dihydroxy–3,6–naphtha-lene disulfonate) colorimetric method, fluoride reacts with the dye lake, dissociating a proportion into a colourless complex anion (ZrF_6^{2-}) and the dye. As the amount of fluoride increases, the colour produced becomes progressively lighter. After preliminary distillation, the distillate is reacted with the zirco-nium-dye lake and measured colorimetrically at 570 nm in a spectrophotometer or at 550 to 580 nm in a filter photometer.

Preparation of standard curve

Prepare fluoride standards
Pipette 5 ml SPADNS and zirconyl-acid reagent
Mix well with standards
Set photometer to zero absorbance
Obtain absorbance readings of standards
Plot a curve of the fluoride-absorbance relationship

Sample pre-treatment

Remove chlorine by adding $NaAsO_2$ solution

Colour development

Adjust 50 ml sample temperature to that used for the
standard curve
Add 5 ml SPADNS solution and zirconyl-acid
Mix well
Read absorbance

Calculation

Figure 6.7   Flow chart of fluoride analysis by SPADNS method.

Method performance

This method is applicable to potable, surface and saline waters as well as domestic and industrial wastewaters. Following distillation to remove interferences, the sample is treated with SPADNS reagent. The loss of colour resulting from the reaction of fluoride with the zirconyl-SPADNS dye is a function of the fluoride concentration. The method covers the range from 0.1 mg l^{-1} to about 1.4 mg l^{-1} (SM 4500F-D). The flow chart for this method is shown in Figure 6.7.

Interference and matrix effects

The SPADNS reagent is more tolerant of interfering materials than other accepted fluoride reagents. The addition of the highly coloured SPADNS reagent must be done with utmost accuracy because the fluoride concentration is measured as a difference of absorbance in the blank and the sample. A small error in reagent addition is the most prominent source of error in this test. Care must be taken to avoid overheating the flask above the level of the solution, i.e. the top of the flame should be maintained so as to heat just the base of the flask.

Sample size
Normally a minimum sample volume of 50 ml is needed for the distillation pre-treatment. The samples collected should be representative and the volumes collected should be sufficient for replicate analysis. Sample preservation is not required but it is recommended to keep the samples cool and to analyse them within 28 days.

Equipment and consumable requirements
Spectrophotometer or filter photometer equipped with a greenish yellow filter is required. The price of the analyser unit is approximately US$ 3,000–10,000. Chemical consumption, which represents the main running cost, is low.

Throughput
Sample preparation is minimal, the time consuming step of analysis being the start up of the equipment. The daily throughput for the equipment is in the range 10–12 samples.

Sample collection, preservation and storage
The samples should be collected in plastic or glass bottles. All bottles must be thoroughly cleaned and rinsed with reagent water. The samples collected should be representative and the volumes collected should be sufficient for replicate analysis. Sample preservation is not required but it is recommended to keep the samples cool and to analyse them within 28 days.

6.6   References

Clesceri, L.S., Greenberg, A.E. and Eaton, A.D. 1998 *Standard Methods for the Examination of Water and Wastewater.* 20th edition, American Public Health Association, American Water Works Association, Water Environment Federation, Washington.

ISO 1990 *8466-1:1990 Water quality — Calibration of analytical methods and estimation of performance characteristics — Part 1: Statistical evaluation of the linear calibration function.* International Standards Organization.

ISO 1992 *10359-1: 1992 Water quality – Determination of fluoride – Part 1: Electrochemical probe method for potable and lightly polluted water.* International Standards Organization.

7

Country data on dental and skeletal fluorosis associated with exposure to fluoride through drinking-water

This chapter provides a synthesis of reported information on fluoride exposure on a country-by-country basis. It outlines the health effects, fluoride levels recorded in drinking-water and also, where details are available, mitigation measures that have been used. Chapters within the main body of the document are cross-referenced as appropriate.

The current WHO guideline value for fluoride in drinking-water is $1.5 \, \text{mg} \, l^{-1}$ (WHO, 2004; see also Chapter 4), and levels above this figure have been defined as elevated for the purposes of this Chapter. However, it should be noted that fluoride toxicity is dependant upon a number of factors, including the quantity of water consumed and exposure to fluoride through other routes. Although fluoride in drinking-water is usually the largest contributor to daily intake, there are other sources of fluoride that may, on occasion, be significant (see Chapter 2). These include, air pollution as a result of burning fluoride-rich coal, certain foods or drinks (such as brick tea) and fluoride supplements.

Health effects related to the exposure to elevated levels of fluoride include dental and skeletal fluorosis (see Chapter 3). A number of indices have been proposed to grade the severity of dental fluorosis and these are outlined in the Appendix.

Waters high in fluoride are mostly calcium-deficient groundwaters in basement aquifers, such as granite and gneiss, in geothermal waters and in some sedimentary basins. Groundwaters with high fluoride concentrations occur in many areas of the world including large parts of Africa, China, the Eastern Mediterranean and southern Asia (India, Sri Lanka). One of the best-known high fluoride belts on land extends along the East African Rift from Eritrea to Malawi. There is another belt from Turkey through Iraq, Iran, Afghanistan, India, northern Thailand and China. The Americas and Japan have similar belts. Where there is sufficient information, the data for each country is divided under a number of self-explanatory headings. The literature review was conducted by searching bibliographic databases (including MEDLINE and POLTOX), bibliographic lists from the collected references and the Internet. Additional information was obtained by consulting individual experts and country or regional representatives. The country-by-country data does not include information on countries that artificially fluoridate their public water supplies.

7.1   Argentina

A survey of groundwater fluoride concentrations in the southeast subhumid pampa of Argentina was conducted by Paoloni et al. (2003). This region, which includes Coronel Dorrego, has a large rural and suburban population that relies on groundwater for drinking-water supplies. Fluoride concentrations occurred in the range 0.9–18.2 mg l^{-1}, with a mean value of 3.8 mg l^{-1}. Only 2.9 per cent of samples analysed were found to be below the guideline value of 1.5 mg l^{-1}.

7.2   Brazil

Some rural communities in Brazil have elevated fluoride levels in their drinking-water supplies. In Paraiba State, for example, which is located in the northeast region, well-derived drinking-water supplies contain 0.1–2.3 mg l^{-1} fluoride (Whitford et al., 1999). In Olho D'Agua (Ceara State), levels of fluoride in drinking-water supplies of 2–3 mg l^{-1} have been recorded, although the concentration varies according to the time of year and depends on rainfall levels (Cortes et al., 1996). Over 62 per cent of children examined in Oldo D'Agua had fluorosis scores of 3 or more based on the Thylstrup-Fejerkov Index (see Appendix).

7.3   Canada

Elevated levels of fluoride in drinking-water have been reported in some communities in Alberta (4.3 mg l^{-1}), Saskatchewan (2.8 mg l^{-1}) and Quebec (2.5 mg l^{-1}) (Droste, 1987; Health Canada, 1993). In Rigolet, Labrador, "moderate" dental fluorosis has been reported associated with exposure to fluoride levels between 0.1–3.8 mg l^{-1} (Ismail and Messer, 1996).

7.4   China

Fluoride-related health effects

In China, fluorosis results from consumption of drinking-water containing elevated fluoride levels, pollution caused by burning fluoride-rich coal and high levels of consumption of brick tea (Wang and Huang, 1995; Cao et al., 1997, 2000; Jin et al., 2000; Toshikazu et al., 2000). Endemic fluorosis is prevalent in China occurring in 29 provinces, municipalities and autonomous regions (Wang and Huang, 1995). The main type of endemic fluorosis in China results from high levels of fluoride in drinking-water (Chen et al., 1997). The geographical distribution is divided into five regions (Sun et al., 2001):

- North-Eastern region (including Heilongjiang, Jilin and Liaoning provinces); Northern and Eastern China (including Hebei, Tianjin, Beijing, Henan, Shandong, Shanxi, Anhui and Jiangsu provinces and municipalities);
- North-West region (including Inner Mongolia, Shaanxi, Ningxia, Qinghai, Gansu and Xinjiang provinces and autonomous region);
- South-Western region (including Sichuan, Yunna, Guangxi, Chongqing and Tibet provinces, municipalities and autonomous regions); and
- other Southern regions (including Guangdong, Fujian, Hunan, Hubei, Jiangxi and Zhejiang provinces).

The highest prevalence of drinking-water-related fluorosis is found in the North-Eastern region.

Dental fluorosis

Dental fluorosis in China has been recognized for some time (Anderson, 1932). It has been estimated that over 26 million people in China suffer from dental fluorosis due to elevated fluoride in their drinking-water, with a further 16.5 million cases of dental fluorosis resulting from coal smoke pollution (Liang et al., 1997). As can be seen from Table 7.1, the prevalence of dental fluorosis is not completely coincident with the fluoride concentration in drinking-water.

Table 7.1   Reported prevalence of dental fluorosis and drinking-water fluoride
concentrations in China

Region	Fluoride concentration in drinking-water (mg l^{-1})	Prevalence of dental fluorosis (%)
Feng county, Jiangsu	9.5	77.3
Pei country, Jiangsu	13	51.9
Shuyang county, Jiangsu	6	75.5
Guannan county, Jiangsu	1.75	47.1
Tianjin	0.8	7.1
Guangdong	0.9	63.2

Sources: Liou (1994); Wang *et al.* (1997); Guo *et al.* (2000)

Table 7.2   Distribution of skeletal fluorosis in China

Region	No. of villages affected	Population affected (10^6)	Cases of skeletal fluorosis (10^6)	Prevalence of skeletal fluorosis (%)
North-East	10,727	6.25	0.147	2.35
Northern and Eastern China	69,558	52.4	0.625	1.20
North-West	32,710	17.6	0.358	2.11
South-West	412	0.51	0.0046	0.90
Southern China	1,395	1.67	0.0037	0.23

Source: Sun *et al.* (2001)

It has been demonstrated that people living in high fluoride drinking-water regions (>4 mg l^{-1}) and consuming a nutrient deficient diet have the highest incidence of dental (and skeletal) fluorosis (Chen *et al.*, 1997; Liang *et al.*, 1997).

Skeletal fluorosis

Over one million cases of skeletal fluorosis are thought to be attributable to drinking-water, with a further million cases due to coal smoke pollution (Liang *et al.*, 1997). Table 7.2 shows the reported distribution of skeletal fluorosis in China (Sun *et al.*, 2001).

Table 7.3   Reported prevalence of skeletal fluorosis associated with
                  increasing drinking-water fluoride concentrations in Jiangsu
                  province, China

Fluoride concentration in drinking-water $(mg \; l^{-1})$	Prevalence of skeletal fluorosis (%)
0.41	0
0.82	1.41
1.02	12.40
1.48	10.16
1.68	7.96
2.60	17.31
3.28	24.84
4.90	26.12
6.40	43.67

Source: Wang *et al.* (1997)

As shown in Table 7.3, there is a significant correlation between the prevalence of skeletal fluorosis and drinking-water fluoride concentration (r = 0.96).
A regression equation between prevalence and fluoride concentration based on
the figures in Table 7.3 (y = 6.55x – 0.48) results in an estimated 0.3 million
cases of skeletal fluorosis in Jiangsu province.

Exposure and fluoride concentrations

Drinking water with high levels of fluoride is widespread in China and has been
seen in all provinces, municipalities and autonomous regions with the exception
of Shanghai, and it has been estimated (Guifan, pers. com.) that there are over
1,200 counties and almost 150,000 villages affected by fluorosis (including coal
pollution derived fluorosis). High fluoride levels in drinking-water are seen
mainly in the arid and semi-arid regions such as Helongjiang, Jilin, Liaoning,
Inner Mongolia, Hebei, Henan, Shanxi, Shaanxi, Ningxia, Gansu and Xinjiang
provinces or autonomous regions (Zheng and Hong, 1988). High fluoride levels
are also seen in hot and cold springs. Hot springs with elevated fluoride concentrations are distributed mainly in Yunnan, Guangdong, Fujian and Taiwan
(Zheng and Hong, 1988; Chen *et al.*, 1997). Fluorosis resulting from elevated
fluoride levels in colds springs is reported mainly in Heilongjiang province.

Fluoride levels in drinking-water can be high, exceeding 3 mg l^{-1}. In the suburbs of Tianjin City, for example, the fluoride content of deep well water has been reported to be 7 mg l^{-1}. In Cangzhou city of Hebei province pressure confined waters have been reported to have fluoride levels between 3 and 8 mg l^{-1} (Zheng and Hong, 1988). In Jilin Province, fluoride concentrations up to 10 mg l^{-1} have been identified and over 50 per cent of samples were found to contain fluoride levels in excess of 2 mg l^{-1} (Zhang et al., 2003). In shallow well water in Pei county (Jiangsu province) levels in excess of 13 mg l^{-1} have been reported (Wang et al., 1997), while hot spring water has been shown to have fluoride levels up to 17 mg l^{-1} (Zheng and Hong, 1988; Guifan, pers. com.).

Mitigation measures

Preventative measures are reported to have been initiated in the 1960s. The principal mitigation strategies include exploitation of deep-seated water, use of river water, reservoir construction and defluoridation, with the use of deep-seated water being one of the most important mitigation strategies (Sun et al., 2000). Since 1980, numerous projects aimed at improving drinking-water quality through the use of defluoridation techniques have been reported as successful (Wang and Huang, 1995). Liang (1998) reported an evaluation of 2000 water engineering projects (amounting to almost 10 per cent of those undertaken) aimed at reducing drinking-water fluoride concentrations. The results demonstrated that the projects were successful, with concentrations of fluoride in drinking-water below 1 mg l^{-1} and decreases seen in the prevalence of dental fluorosis. According to Sun et al. (2000) an overall coverage rate of safe water supplies of 60–70 per cent has been provided using deep-seated wells in the endemic fluorosis areas.

7.5   Eritrea

Fluoride levels in drinking-water were not considered, generally, to present a large risk of fluorosis. The mean recorded fluoride levels in Eritrea are 0.99 mg l^{-1} in the Northern Red Sea, 0.16 mg l^{-1} in Zoba Gash-Barka, 0.27 mg l^{-1} in the Southern Red Sea, 2.10 mg l^{-1} in the Northern Red Sea, 0.16 mg l^{-1} in Zoba Anseba and 0.56 mg l^{-1} in Zoba Debub (Water Resources Department, Eritrea, unpublished report, 1999). Mottling of the teeth has been observed in children from eight villages around Keren (Srikanth et al., 2002). This observation led to an investigation of the fluoride levels in the drinking-water serving the affected villages. Srikanth et al. (2002) found that, with the exception of Wasdenba (with a fluoride level of 1.2 mg l^{-1}), all of the sources in the other seven villages had fluoride levels greater than 1.5 mg l^{-1} (ranging 2.02–3.73 mg l^{-1}). The authors estimated from these findings that around 15,000 people were at risk from high fluoride levels.

7.6   Ethiopia

Fluoride-related health effects

Dental fluorosis
Olsson (1979) reported dental fluorosis in 99 per cent of 239, 6–7 year-old, children examined living in Wonji and Awassa in the Rift Valley. The fluoride concentration in Wonji and Awassa was 12.4 and 3.5 mg l^{-1}, respectively (Olsson, 1979). A study conducted by Haimanot *et al.* (1987) found dental fluorosis in more than 80 per cent of sampled children resident in the Rift Valley since birth (1,221 out of 1,456). The maximum prevalence was seen in the 10–14 year old age-group and 32 per cent of the children showed severe dental mottling. Males were affected more than females (Haimanot *et al.*, 1987). Wondwossen *et al.* (2004) examined dental fluorosis (and caries) in children living in two villages in the Wonji Shoa sugar estate. Fluoride levels in the two villages were markedly different (village A: 0.3–2.2 mg l^{-1}; village K: 10–14 mg l^{-1}). The prevalence of dental fluorosis (a score of 1 or more using the Thylstrup-Fejerskov index – see Appendix) was 91.8 per cent in village A and 100 per cent in village K. The prevalence of severe dental fluorosis (a score of 5 or greater), however, was 11 per cent in village A and 60 per cent in village K.

Skeletal fluorosis
Skeletal fluorosis was first reported in Ethiopia in 1973 in the Wonji Shoa sugar estates in the Ethiopian Rift Valley (Lester, 1974). Three areas, Wonji-Shoa, Alemtena and Samiberta, have been identified as having cases of skeletal fluorosis. The highest incidence was found at the Wonji-Shoa sugar estates, where a linear relationship was observed between the development of crippling fluorosis, fluoride concentration in drinking-water supplies and period of exposure. The first cases of skeletal fluorosis appeared among workers on the estates (98 per cent males) who had been consuming water with fluoride content of more than 8 mg l^{-1} for over 10 years. Between 1976 and 1984, 530 workers were retired from Wonji-Shoa at the age of 45–50 years because of inability to perform their physically strenuous jobs. Among these workers, 46 per cent were found to have skeletal fluorosis. In August 1984, a medical board examined 300 persons from Wonji-Shoa with a presumptive diagnosis of skeletal fluorosis after complaints of pains and aches in the joints, limitation of movement, and progressive kyphosis (excessive outward curvature of the spine). Radiological

evidence of skeletal fluorosis was found in 65 per cent of the 300 persons examined and 30 (10 per cent) had crippling fluorosis (Haimanot *et al.*, 1987).

Exposure and fluoride concentrations

The region of the Rift Valley in Ethiopia varies between 500 and 1,800 metres above sea level, and is hot and dry, with a mean temperature of 23 °C (range 15 °C to 38 °C). The Wonji Shoa sugar estates and Metahara Sugar Estate are the major agro-industrial establishments in the Rift Valley, with a population of 31,000 and 25,000 respectively. A study conducted in 16 large farms, villages and towns in the Ethiopian Rift Valley between 1977 and 1985 found that the fluoride level of drinking-water collected from wells there ranged from 1.2 to 36.0 mg l^{-1} (mean 10.0 mg l^{-1}). The sugar estates, which had the highest population densities, generally had fluoride levels far in excess of the WHO guideline value, with Wonji-Shoa having levels between 3.7 and 17.0 mg l^{-1}, and Metahara 2.4 to 7.0 mg l^{-1} (Haimanot *et al.*, 1987). Initial results from a programme to measure fluoride in wells from all over Ethiopia found that, from the 138 wells tested, 33 per cent had fluoride concentration greater than 1.5 mg l^{-1}; the maximum level detected was over 11.5 mg l^{-1} (Reimann *et al.*, 2003). The high fluoride concentrations were all clustered in wells from the centre of the Ethiopian part of the Rift valley, which suggests a hydrothermal origin for the fluoride.

Mitigation measures

In the early 1970s, defluoridated water supplies were reported to have been available in all factories in the area, following the recognition of this problem (Haimanot *et al.* 1987). It would seem, however, that the defluoridation plants do not always operate, because a study looking at fluoride intake in children in the Wonji Shoa sugar estate found levels of fluoride of 14.4 mg l^{-1} in well water from one of the villages (Malde *et al.*, 2004).

7.7   Germany

Two cases of severe dental fluorosis were identified in 1998 in school children living in the Muenster region of Germany. Both cases occurred in one household and resulted from excessive fluoride consumption both through supplements and elevated levels in the drinking-water supply (Queste *et al.*, 2001). The discovery of these cases led to an examination of other rural wells in the region, a large number of which were found to have elevated fluoride levels with concentrations up to 8.8 mg l^{-1}. Grafe and Dominok (1978) reported skeletal fluorosis in an 80-year-old man, whose drinking-water was contaminated by the effluent from a local fluoride plant.

7.8   India

Fluoride-related health effects
A total of 17 (out of 32) States are reported to have endemic fluorosis in India (FRRDF, 1999; Yadav et al., 1999). In 1987, it was estimated that 25 million people were suffering from fluorosis (FRRDF, 1999).

Dental fluorosis
The prevalence of dental fluorosis has been investigated in Rajasthan by Choubisa et al. (1997). Prevalence rates were observed in 15 tribal villages with fluoride concentrations of 0.3–10.8 mg l^{-1}. At mean fluoride concentrations of 1.4 and 6 mg l^{-1}, dental fluorosis was seen in 25.6 per cent and 84.4 per cent of school children (< 16 years) and 23.9 per cent and 96.9 per cent of adults respectively. Kodali et al. (1994) reported dental mottling in 76 per cent of children in the 5–10 year age group and 84 per cent of children in the 10–15 year age group in Kodabakshupally, Sarampet and Sivannagudem. Yadav and Lata (2003) examined the prevalence of dental fluorosis at lower drinking-water fluoride concentrations (mean concentrations between 1.93 and 2.14 mg l^{-1}) in the Jhajjar district, Haryana. Over 50 per cent of the children examined were found to be affected by dental fluorosis. Reddy and Prasad (2003) reported dental fluorosis levels of 43 per cent in the Anantapur district of Andhra Pradesh, where drinking-water fluoride concentrations ranged between 1.2 and 2.1 mg l^{-1}.

Skeletal fluorosis
Endemic skeletal fluorosis was reported from India in the 1930s. It was observed first in Andhra Pradesh bullocks used for ploughing, when farmers noticed the bullocks inability to walk, apparently due to painful and stiff joints. Several years later the same disease was observed in humans (Short et al., 1937). Choubisa et al. (1997) examined the prevalence of skeletal fluorosis in Rajasthan in adults exposed to mean fluoride levels of 1.4 and 6 mg l^{-1}. At 1.4 mg l^{-1} over 4 per cent of adults were reported to be affected, while at 6 mg l^{-1}, 63 per cent of adults were reported to be affected. The prevalence was found to be higher in males and increased with increasing fluoride levels and age. In Andhra Pradesh, Reddy and Prasad (2003) found skeletal fluorosis affecting between 0.2 and 1 per cent of the population examined, where the maximum drinking-water fluoride concentration was 2.1 mg l^{-1}.

Exposure, fluorosis and fluoride concentrations
At least 17 States are affected by elevated fluoride levels in drinking-water, namely; Andhra Pradesh, Assam, Bihar, Delhi, Gujarat, Haryana, Jammu and Kashmir, Kamataka, Kerala, Madhya Pradesh, Maharashtra, Orissa, Punjab,

Table 7.4   Fluoride concentrations reported in groundwaters of India

Region/State	Fluoride concentration (mg l^{-1})	Maximum severity of fluorosis observed
North-West India	0.4 – 19	Severe
Central India	0.2 – 10	Moderate
South India	0.2 – 20	Severe
Deccan Province	0.4 – 8	Moderate

Sources: Agarwal *et al.* (1997); Yadav *et al.* (1999)

Rajasthan, Tamil Nadu, Uttar Pradesh and West Bengal. These have been progressively identified since the first report by Short *et al.* (1937), with Assam being the most recently identified State with high fluoride levels associated with endemic fluorosis. Not all States are equally affected and the number of districts with endemic fluorosis within each State varies (FRRDF, 1999). Nine out of eighteen districts in West Bengal were recently identified as having fluoride contaminated groundwater (Ministry of Water Resources, 2004). It has been estimated that the total population consuming drinking-water containing elevated levels of fluoride is over 66 million (FRRDF, 1999). The distribution of fluoride in Indian groundwaters is shown in Table 7.4.

In Rajasthan, fluoride concentrations have been found to vary between 0.6 mg l^{-1} and 69.7 mg l^{-1} (Gupta, 1999). In Haryana, the highest fluoride concentration was found in the village of Karoli and was recorded at 48 mg l^{-1} (Kim-Farley, pers. com.). Meenakshi *et al.* (2004) reported fluoride levels of between 0.3 and 6.9 mg l^{-1} in four villages in the Jind district of Haryana.

Mitigation measures

Formal mitigation measures were undertaken from 1987, when the Government of India made a commitment to provide safe water to the rural community (i.e. those most affected by fluorosis). Since 1987, numerous programmes aimed at fully identifying the problem, along with developing fluoride removal tech-niques have been implemented (FRRDF, 1999). In the Dungarpur district of Rajasthan, activated alumina and Nalgonda defluoridation are practised. Defluoridation kits have been distributed at household level under the sponsorship of UNICEF and active community participation has been observed with the result that it has been reported that the ongoing Fluorosis Mitigation Programme is sustainable (Vaish and Vaish, 2000). In Andhra Pradesh the use of check dams, to dilute fluoride concentrations in groundwater, has been investigated (Bhagavan and Raghu, 2005). The check dams, which are rainwater harvesting structures, are designed to provide artificial recharge of groundwater. In over 50 per cent of cases, the check dams were found to reduce fluoride concentrations in groundwater.

7.9 Indonesia

Fluoride concentrations in drinking-water have been investigated in the Asembagus coastal plain, in the north-eastern part of Java (Heikens *et al.*, 2005). Fluoride concentrations in well water were <0.1–4.2 mg l^{-1}. The wells with the highest fluoride concentrations were those closest to the river Banyuputih, which is contaminated with effluent from the hyperacid crater lake of the Ijen volcano. The river water was found to contain an average fluoride level of 9.5 mg l^{-1}, although this was found to fluctuate between 5.5 and 14.2 mg l^{-1}.

7.10 Israel

Milgalter *et al.* (1974) found natural fluoride levels in drinking-water of up to 3 mg l^{-1} in the Negev desert region.

7.11 Japan

Dental fluorosis was observed in children of the Ikeno district in the Aichi prefecture in the 1970s, following the unintentional supply of drinking-water containing up to 7.8 mg l^{-1} fluoride since 1960 (Ishii and Suckling, 1991). On discovery of the high fluoride levels, an alternative supply with a fluoride level of 0.2 mg l^{-1} was provided.

Tsutsui *et al.* (2000) examined the prevalence of dental fluorosis in Japanese communities exposed to naturally occurring fluoride up to 1.4 mg l^{-1}. A total of 1,060, 10–12 year-old, lifetime residents were examined. The prevalence of dental fluorosis was found to increase as fluoride levels increased, ranging from 1.7 per cent at 0.2–0.4 mg l^{-1} up to 15.4 per cent in the group exposed to 1.1–1.4 mg l^{-1}.

Table 7.5   Reported prevalences of dental fluorosis in Kenya

| | | Distribution of signs of dental fluorosis (%) | | | | | | |
| | | Absent | | Present | | | | Preval -ence |
Race	No.	Normal	Questionable	Very mild	Mild	Moderate	Severe	(%)
European	922	61.3	15.7	13.4	6.4	2.3	0.9	23.0
Asian	626	30.4	11.7	17.5	28.6	5.7	6.1	57.9
African	3,014	46.4	15.7	17.9	10.8	5.5	3.7	37.9

Classified according to the degree of affliction. Prevalence in all racial groups: 39.6 per cent
Source: Williamson (1953)

7.12 Kenya

Fluoride-related health effects

Dental fluorosis

Nevill and Brass (1953) examined 1,202 European children between the ages of 7 and 14 living in Kenya. According to this study, a total of 30 per cent of the children were showing some degree of dental fluorosis. Williamson (1953) also examined levels of dental fluorosis and the incidence is shown in Table 7.5.

Dental fluorosis is reported in the Northern Frontier (Turkana), North-West Kenya, South Rift Valley and Central and Eastern Regions (Fendall and Grounds, 1965). A survey of 1,307 Asian and African school children found that 67 per cent of Asian children and 47 per cent of African children were affected. The degree of dental fluorosis was reported to be more severe among Asian children, and it was speculated that this could have been related to their vegetarian diet (Fendall and Grounds, 1965). Manji *et al.* (1986a) examined 110 children living in an area of Kenya with 2 mg l^{-1} fluoride in the water and found that all the children examined exhibited dental fluorosis.

Dental fluorosis has also been identified in an area with a relatively low fluoride concentration. Manji *et al.* (1986b) examined 160 children living in an area where the fluoride concentration ranged between 0.54 and 0.93 mg l^{-1} and showed that the prevalence of enamel changes was 93.8 per cent. Severe dental fluorosis (TFI 5 or more – see Appendix) was seen in over 33 per cent of the children.

Altitude may have an effect on the level of dental fluorosis. According to Manji *et al.* (1986c) in low fluoride drinking-water zones (<0.5 mg l^{-1}) 36 per cent of the children at sea level had dental fluorosis, compared with 78 per cent at

1,500 m and 100 per cent at 2,400 m. In higher fluoride zones (0.5–1.0 mg l^{-1}), 71 per cent had dental fluorosis at sea level as compared to almost 94 per cent at 1,500 m.

Skeletal fluorosis

Fendall and Grounds (1965) reported a single case of skeletal fluorosis in a European living in Kenya. He had been exposed to borehole water containing 18–29 mg l^{-1} fluoride for a period of six years.

Exposure and fluoride concentrations

The fluoride content of borehole water varies considerably across different bore-holes (even when in close proximity) and may also show temporal variations between the same borehole (Nair and Manji, 1982). The highest concentrations of fluoride in groundwater are reported to occur in the peri-urban areas of Nairobi, in the Rift Valley around Nakuru, Naivasha and Mount Kenya, and near the northern frontier. Local pockets of intermediate concentrations of 2–20 mg l^{-1} have been reported throughout the country. According to Fendall and Grounds (1965) excess fluoride in surface water occurs in Lakes Rudolph (12 mg l^{-1}), Hannington (1,100 mg l^{-1}), Baringo (6 mg l^{-1}), Nakuru (2,400 mg l^{-1}), Magadi and elsewhere. Nair *et al.* (1984) reported concentrations of fluoride up to 1,640 mg l^{-1} and 2,800 mg l^{-1} in lakes Elmentaita and Nukuru respectively. In a study of over 1,000 groundwater samples taken nationally over 60 per cent exceeded 1 mg l^{-1}, 20 per cent exceeded 5 mg l^{-1} and 12 per cent exceeded 8 mg l^{-1}. The volcanic areas of the Nairobi Rift Valley and Central Provinces had the highest concentrations, with maximum groundwater fluoride concentrations reaching 50 mg l^{-1} (Nair *et al.*, 1984).

7.13 Mexico

Fluoride-related health effects

Fluorosis is considered to be a largely unrecognized environmental health problem in Mexico (Díaz-Barriga *et al.*, 1997a).

Dental fluorosis

In the city of San Luis Potosi, 98 per cent of children exposed to fluoride drinking-water concentrations of greater than 2 mg l^{-1} were reported to exhibit signs of dental fluorosis (Grimaldo *et al.*, 1995). Bottled juice and bottled water containing high levels of fluoride were also felt to contribute to the levels of dental fluorosis in San Luis Potosi, and help explain the high levels of fluorosis in children not exposed to elevated levels in their drinking-water supply (Díaz-Barriga *et al.*, 1997b).

Skeletal fluorosis
No references could be found documenting cases of skeletal fluorosis although, as pointed out by Díaz-Barriga *et al.* (1997a), the exposure to elevated levels of fluoride began in the late 1960s. Results of X-ray and densitometry tests conducted on cases possibly showing early signs of skeletal fluorosis were inconclusive (Calderón *et al.*, 1995).

Exposure and fluoride concentrations
Diaz-Barriga *et al.* (1997a) estimated that approximately 5 million people may be exposed to elevated levels of fluoride in their drinking-water supplies. Mean fluoride concentrations in urban locations ranged from 1.5 to 2.8 mg l^{-1}, although individual sources were recorded as having concentrations up to 7.8 mg l^{-1} (Hermosillo in Sonara State). In rural locations a similar pattern occurred with mean levels between 0.9 and 4.5 mg l^{-1} and the highest recorded concentration of 8 mg l^{-1} (Abasolo in Guanajuato State). States with elevated fluoride levels included Aguascalientes, Chihuahua, Coahuila, Durango, Guanajuato, San Luis Potosi and Sonora (Díaz-Barriga *et al.*, 1997a). In the city of Durango, it has been estimated that almost 95 per cent of the residents were exposed to fluoride concentrations in drinking-water greater than 2 mg l^{-1} (Ortiz *et al.*, 1998). Hurtado and Gardea-Torresdey (2004) reported high levels of fluoride from drinking-water from the Los Altos de Jalisco region. Over 40 per cent of the municipalities had fluoride concentrations greater than 1.5 mg l^{-1}. Three of the cities in the region had particularly elevated levels, most notably Teocaltiche (up to 18.5 mg l^{-1}).

7.14 Niger

Over 400 children, ranging in age from 15 months to 14 years were reported to have skeletal fluorosis in Tibiri, with 68 per cent of the illness being seen in 5 year-olds. Bony lesions were first observed in 1988. This led to analysis of the water and the discovery of high fluoride levels (4.7–6.6 mg l^{-1}). Mitigation measures were undertaken, with water being brought in from a neighbouring area, and Niger's water company confirmed that the level of fluoride had fallen to 1.6 mg l^{-1} (Arji, 2001; Ziegler, 2002).

7.15 Nigeria

A literature search revealed only one study into the occurrence of dental fluorosis in Nigeria (Wongdem *et al.*, 2000). A total of 475 people aged 5 and over, who were either born in Langtang town or had lived there for a minimum of 5 years, were examined. Enamel status was assessed for mottling using a modified version of Dean's classification (see Appendix). There was a 26.1 per cent prevalence rate of enamel fluorosis in the Langtang town area, with 20.6 per cent of the cases classified as mild and 5.5 per cent as severe. The highest prevalence was seen among 10 to 19 year olds. A follow-up study to determine the fluoride concentrations in Langtang town, found that levels ranged between 0.5 and 3.96 mg l^{-1} with the highest levels being found in stream sources (Wongdem *et al.*, 2001).

7.16 Norway

In Norway more than 80 per cent of the population presently receive drinking-water from surface water sources. As surface water fluoride concentrations are very low, Norway has traditionally been considered a low-fluoride area, and dental fluorosis was not considered to be a problem. However, due to increasing regional environmental pollution and microbiological problems, Norwegian authorities have been looking for alternative drinking-water sources and the Norwegian Geological Survey has been actively promoting the use of groundwater, estimating that by the year 2000 about 30 per cent of the population would have been supplied from underground water sources.

Approximately 100,000 private drinking-water wells were reported to be in use in Norway and several thousand new wells were being drilled every year (Bardsen and Bjorvatn, 1998; Bardsen *et al.*, 1999). Investigations showed that groundwater could contain high concentrations of fluoride. A study from the county of Hordaland, for example, reported fluoride concentrations in groundwater in the range of 0.02–9.48 mg l^{-1} (Bardsen *et al.*, 1999). Dental fluorosis has been reported among lifelong consumers of moderate to high fluoride-containing groundwater (0.5–8.0 mg l^{-1}) (Bardsen *et al.*, 1999).

7.17 Pakistan

Generally, the majority of drinking-water sources in Pakistan are reported to contain acceptable levels of fluoride, with 84 per cent containing less than 0.7 mg l^{-1} (Ayyaz *et al.*, 2002). However, this may not be true in areas of northern Pakistan, as has been shown for Kheshki and Naranji, northeast of Peshawar (Shah and Danishwar, 2003). Levels of fluoride in spring and stream sources of between 8 and 13.52 mg l⁻¹ have been reported for Naranji and the surrounding area (Shah and Danishwar, 2003).

Fluoride Action Network (2001) reported an incident in a village close to Lahore, where skeletal fluorosis was seen in a number of children as a result of fluoride in factory waste contaminating the local water supply.

7.18 Saudi Arabia

In the Hail region, over 90 per cent of 2,355 rural children examined and aged 12–15 years were reported to show dental fluorosis, and a strong association ($p < 0.001$) was seen between fluoride level (0.5–2.8 mg l⁻¹) in well water used for drinking and the severity of dental fluorosis (Akpata *et al.*, 1997). Mecca (with a fluoride concentration up to 2.5 mg l⁻¹) was also reported to be an area with endemic fluorosis (Al-Khateeb *et al.*, 1991; Akpata *et al.*, 1997).

7.19 Senegal

Fluoride concentrations in drinking-water at Kaffrine, Gossas, Guinguinéo, Foundiougne (in the Sine Saloum region) and Darou Rahmane Fall (in the Diourbel region) were found to be 1.1, 2.6, 3.9, 4.6, and 7.4 mg l⁻¹, respectively. Prevalence of dental fluorosis among the children at Kaffrine, Gossas, Guinguinéo, and Foundiougne was 68.5, 85.3, 93.7 and 100 per cent, respectively. About 30 per cent and 60 per cent of the children in Guinguinéo and Darou Rahmane Fall, respectively, were reported to have severely discoloured brownish-black teeth (Brouwer *et al.*, 1988).

7.20 South Africa

Fluoride-related health effects

Mauguhan-Brown (1935), Staz (1938) and Abrahams (1946) reported the presence of fluorosis amongst children in high fluoride areas of South Africa. Ockerse (1944, 1949) identified 803 endemic fluorosis areas in South Africa, mostly the North Western, Western and Karoo Regions of Cape Province, Western and Central Free State, and Northern, Eastern and Western areas of Transvaal.

Dental fluorosis

In the Western Bushveld areas, which are known to have endemic dental fluorosis, about 300,000 people drink water with fluoride concentrations above 0.7 mg l^{-1}. Dental fluorosis in both children and adults is clearly manifested in many villages (McCaffrey and Willis, 1997). A study on the perceptions of fluorosis conducted in the northern Cape (Chikte *et al.*, 2001) demonstrated that fluoride concentrations should be kept below 0.7 mg l^{-1} in order to minimize the risk of dental fluorosis. This was based on a study of teeth from 694 children living in three areas with differing fluoride concentrations categorized as suboptimal (0.4–0.6 mg l^{-1}), optimal (0.99–1.1 mg l^{-1}) and supra-optimal (1.70–2.70 mg l^{-1}). Even in the suboptimal fluoride area children showed signs of dental fluorosis, with 19 per cent of the group considered to be experiencing moderate or severe fluorosis. In the supra-optimal category, 45 per cent of children exhibited severe fluorosis. Grobler *et al.* (2001) examined the level of dental fluorosis in 282 children living in Sanddrif (0.19 mg l^{-1} fluoride), Kuboes (0.48 mg l^{-1} fluoride) and Leeu Gamka (3 mg l^{-1} fluoride). The prevalence of fluorosis (scores greater than 2 using Deans index – see Appendix) was 47 per cent in Sanddrif, 50 per cent in Kuboes and 95 per cent in Leeu Gamka. Except for one child in Kuboes, severe fluorosis (a score of 5 or greater) was only observed in Leeu Gamka with 30 per cent of the children affected. Ncube and Schutte (2005) reported levels of dental fluorosis in Free State, Western Cape, KwaZulu-Natal and North-West Provinces. The highest level of fluorosis (classified as slight to heavy) was in the North-West Province, where up to 73 per cent of children were affected.

Skeletal fluorosis

Cases of severe skeletal fluorosis in adults have been reported in villages in the Western Bushveld area (McCaffrey and Willis, 1997).

Exposure and fluoride concentrations

High fluoride groundwater is found inside the Pilanesberg Alkaline Igneous Complex (mean 3.7 mg l^{-1}) and very high fluoride concentrations (mean 57 mg l^{-1}) are found around the perimeter. High fluoride concentrations in groundwater are also found in the Nebo Granite and the mineralized Lebowa Granite. It is suggested that the cause of most high fluoride concentrations in groundwater is the dissolution of fluoride bearing minerals in bedrock and soil. Microscopic study of thin sections of common rock types from the area showed that fluorite, mica and hornblende were the most common fluoride bearing minerals (McCaffrey, 1995). A large part of the population in the Karoo, Northern Cape and North West Province drink water from boreholes due to the low level of annual rainfall (Moola, 1996). Grobler *et al.* (2001) noted that heavy rainfall could markedly decrease the fluoride levels in drinking-water in South Africa.

7.21 Spain

Areas in Tenerife, mainly in the north of the island, have high levels of fluoride in drinking-water and cases of fluorosis have been observed. In the affected areas of La Guancha, San Juan de la Rambla and Icod de los Vinos mean fluoride concentrations varied between 2.50 and 4.59 mg l^{-1} (Hardisson *et al.*, 2001).

7.22 Sri Lanka

Problems relating to elevated levels of fluoride in drinking-water in Sri Lanka are relatively recent and reflect the increase in the number of tubewells, particularly in the "Dry Zone" in the North Central Province, where levels of fluoride up to 10 mg l^{-1} have been reported (Dissanayake, 1996). Defluoridation, using charcoal and charred bone meal, has been introduced in some areas (Dissanayake, 1996; Saparamadu, 2000).

7.23 Sudan

Fluorosis was reported in the course of an investigation into health and nutrition at Abu Deleig in the Butana desert, 105 miles east of Khartoum, in December 1952. Many cases were seen also at Jevel Geili, an encampment 30 miles to the south, but none at Wad Hssuna, a large village about 30 miles west of Abu Deleig. The fluoride content of drinking-water in Abu Deleig and Jebel Gaili was recorded as between 0.65 and 3.20 mg l^{-1}. Examination of 134 schoolboys living in Abu Deleig showed the total incidence of dental fluorosis to be 60.4 per cent (Smith *et al.*, 1953).

7.24 Thailand

Drinking water fluoride levels have been found to exceed 10 mg l^{-1} in some parts of Thailand. Northern and western Thailand were considered the most likely to have high fluoride levels and it has been estimated that approximately 1 per cent of natural water sources contain levels greater than 2 mg l^{-1} (Prasertsom, 1998). In northern Thailand high fluoride levels may be associated with geothermal sources of water (Noppakun *et al.*, 2000). The highest level of fluoride recorded by Chuckpaiwong *et al.* (2000) was 0.92 mg l^{-1} and groundwater sources were found to contain the highest levels of fluoride.

7.25 Turkey

There are a number of areas in Turkey where drinking-water fluoride concentrations can be very high, especially in the middle and eastern part of Turkey. In Denizli-Sarayköy and Çaldiran Plain levels can reach 13.7 mg l^{-1}, while in Eskişehir and Isparta levels from 1.9 to 7.5 mg l^{-1} and from 3.8 to 4.9 mg l^{-1} respectively, have been reported (Azbar and Türkman, 2000).

7.26 Uganda

Dental fluorosis has been seen in the Rift Valley area of western Uganda (Rwenyonyi *et al.*, 1998). A number of studies (Rwenyonyi *et al.*, 1998, 2000) have examined the determinants of dental fluorosis in children in this region, comparing low fluoride areas (0.5 mg l^{-1}) with high fluoride areas (2.5 mg l^{-1}). Altitude was found to affect both the prevalence and severity of fluorosis in both high and low fluoride areas. In the high fluoride area, the severity of fluorosis was also found to increase with age.

7.27 United Republic of Tanzania

Fluoride-related health effects

Dental fluorosis
Grech (1966), reported that all the 119 children examined in Maji ya Chai aged between 9 and 13 years were found to have dental fluorosis; 87.4 per cent of them to a severe degree. They had lived their entire lives in this area, consuming only the local spring or river water. The river fluoride concentration was found to be 18.6 mg l^{-1}. Of people examined around Arusha and Moshi, between 83 and 95 per cent exhibited dental fluorosis. Awadia *et al.* (1999) found that in Arusha the prevalence and severity of fluorosis was greater in non-vegetarians (fluorosis – 95 per cent, severe fluorosis – 35 per cent) than in vegetarians (fluorosis – 67 per cent, severe fluorosis – 21 per cent).

Skeletal fluorosis
Skeletal manifestations have been reported around Arusha (Grech, 1966; Mosha, 1984). Endemic fluorosis is a public health problem in some parts of the United

Table 7.6   Fluoride level in the United Republic of Tanzanian water sources

Water source	Fluoride concentration (mg l^{-1})
Maji ya Chai River	12 – 13
Pond waters and Kitefu area	61 – 65
Engare Nanyuki River	21 – 26
Lake Momella	up to 690
Mbulu area springs	up to 99

Source: Mjengera (1988) cited in Kaseva (1993)

Republic of Tanzania, namely: Arusha, Moshi, Singida and Shinyanga regions. According to Mosha (1984), it is particularly severe around Arusha situated in the Rift Valley (on the foot hills of Mount Meru, which has approximately 135,000 inhabitants) and Moshi (on the foot hills of Mount Kilimanjaro).

Exposure and fluoride concentrations
In the African Rift System, fluoride-rich waters are associated with volcanic activity. Due to high temperatures and high pH levels, surface waters (as well as groundwater) contain high fluoride concentrations. The fluoride levels recorded from some water sources in the United Republic of Tanzania are shown in Table 7.6. The majority of the Tanzanian population obtain their drinking-water from lakes, rivers or springs (Mosha, 1984).

Awadia *et al.* (2000) reported similar levels of dental fluorosis in two areas with marked differences in fluoride drinking-water levels (0.2 mg l^{-1} and 3.6 mg l^{-1}). It was suggested that the high level of fluorosis seen in the low fluoride area may be at least partly explained by the use of high fluoride foods, such as magadi, in weaning preparations.

Mitigation measures
The Nalgonda technique (as outlined in section 5.4) was first adopted for defluoridation in the United Republic of Tanzania in 1974 (Mosha, 1984).

7.28 United States of America
Historically, dental fluorosis was quite widespread in the USA. Originally the problem was termed "mottled enamel" or, local to Colorado Springs, as

"Colorado brown strain". In 1930, the link was made between mottled enamel and high levels of fluoride in drinking-water supplies (2.0–13.7 mg l^{-1}) and the term fluorosis was adopted (MMWR, 1999). A system for estimating the severity of dental fluorosis (see Appendix) known as Deans Index was developed (Dean and Dixon, 1935; Dean and Elvove, 1939). Dean also conducted extensive observational studies to assess the prevalence of fluorosis in the USA (Dean, 1933). Arizona, Arkansas, California, Colorado, Idaho, Illinois, Iowa, Kansas, Minnesota, Nevada, New Mexico, North Carolina, North Dakota, Oklahoma, Oregon, South Carolina, South Dakota, Texas, Utah and Virginia were also reported to have areas with endemic fluorosis (Dean, 1933). These studies also led to the realization of the link between low levels of fluoride and high prevalence of caries (Dean, 1938, 1945), which culminated in the recommendation that levels of fluoride in water be adjusted to between 0.7–1.2 mg l^{-1} (Public Health Service, 1962) and the adoption of widespread fluoridation.

Driscoll *et al.* (1983) noted that more than 700 communities in the USA were thought to have water supplies that contained at least twice the recommended optimum level of fluoride (i.e. 2.4 mg l^{-1} and above). They found mean fluoride concentrations in Illinois between 1.06 and 4.07 mg l^{-1}. In a study in Texas (Segreto *et al.*, 1984), fluoride concentrations varied between 0.3 and 4.3 mg l^{-1}. At the highest fluoride concentration only 5.2 per cent of children were considered to have normal teeth or questionable mottling.

7.29 References

Abrahams, L.C. 1946 The masticatory apparatus of Calvinia and Namaqualand in the North Western Cape of the Union of South Africa. *Journal of the Dental Association of South Africa*, **1**, 4–9.

Agarwal, V., Vaish, A.K. and Vaish, P. 1997 Ground water quality: Focus on fluoride and fluorosis in Rajasthan. *Current Science*, **73**(9), 743–746.

Akpata, E.S., Fakiha, Z. and Khan, N. 1997 Dental fluorosis in 12–15-year-old rural children exposed to fluorides from well drinking water in the Hail region of Saudi Arabia. *Community Dentistry and Oral Epidemiology*, **25** (4), 324–327.

Al-Khateeb, T.L., Al-Marasafi, A.I. and O'Mullane, D.M. 1991 Caries prevalence and treatment need amongst children in an Arabian community. *Community Dentistry and Oral Epidemiology*, **19**, 277–280.

Anderson, B.G. 1932 An endemic center of mottled enamel in China. *Journal of Dental Research,* **12**, 591–593.

Arji, S. 2001 Health-Niger: Hundreds of children poisoned by tap water. Inter Press Service (http://www.oneworld.net/ips2/jan01/17_44_015.htm).

Awadia, A.K., Birkeland, J.M., Haugejorden, O. and Bjorvatn, K. 2000 An attempt to explain why Tanzanian children drinking water containing 0.2 or 3.6 mg fluoride per liter exhibit a similar level of dental fluorosis. *Clinical Oral Investigations,* **4**(4), 238–244.

Awadia, A.K., Haugejorden, O., Bjorvatn, K. and Birkeland, J.M. 1999 Vegetarianism and dental fluorosis among children in a high fluoride area of northern Tanzania. International *Journal of Paediatric Dentistry*, **9**(1), 3–11.

Ayyaz, A.K., Whelton, H., O'Mullane, D. 2002 A map of natural fluoride in drinking water in Pakistan. *International Dentistry Journal,* **52** (4), 291–297.

Azbar, N. and Türkman, A. 2000 Defluoridation in drinking water. *Water Science and Technology,* **42**(1–2), 403–407.

Bardsen, A. and Bjorvatn, K. 1998 Risk periods in the development of dental fluorosis. *Clinical Oral Investigations*, **2**(4), 155–160.

Bardsen, A., Klock, K.S. and Bjorvatn, K. 1999 Dental fluorosis among persons exposed to high- and low-fluoride drinking water in western Norway. *Community Dentistry and Oral Epidemiology,* **27**(4), 259–267.

Bhagavan, S.V.B.K. and Raghu, V. 2005 Utility of check dams in dilution of fluoride concentrations in ground water and the resultant analysis of blood serum and urine of villagers, Anantapur district, Andhra Pradesh, India. *Environmental Geochemistry and Health,* **27**, 97–108.

Brouwer, I.D., Dirks, O.B., De-Bruin, A. and Hautvast, J.G.A.J. 1988 Unsuitability of World Health Organization Guidelines for fluoride concentrations in drinking water in Senegal. *Lancet*, Jan 30, 223–225.

Calderón, J., Romieu, I., Grimaldo, M., Hernández, H. and Díaz-Barriga, F. 1995 Endemic fluorosis in San Luis Potosí, Mexico. II Identification of risk factors associated with occupational exposure to fluoride. *Fluoride,* **28**, 203–208.

Cao, J., Zhao, Y and Liu, J. 1997 Brick tea consumption as the cause of dental fluorosis among children from Mongol, Kasak and Yugu populations in China. *Food Chemistry and Toxicology,* **35**(8), 827–833.

Cao, J., Zhao, Y., Liu, J., Xirao, R. and Danzneg, S. 2000 [Environmental fluorine level in Tibet] *Ying Yong Sheng Tai Xue Bao,* **11**(5), 777–779. Article in Chinese.

Chen, Y.C., Lin, M,Q., Xia, Y.D., Gan, W.M., Min, D. and Chen, C. 1997 Nutritional survey in dental fluorosis-afflicted areas. *Fluoride,* **30**(2), 77–80.

Chikte, U.M., Louw, A.J. and Stander, I. 2001 Perceptions of fluorosis in northern Cape communities. *Journal of the South African Dental Association*, **56**(11), 528–532.

Choubisa, S.L., Choubisa, D.K., Joshi, S.C. and Choubisa, L. 1997 Fluorosis in some tribal villages of Dungarpur district of Rajasthan, India. *Fluoride*, **30**(4), 223–228.

Chuckpaiwong, S., Nakornchai, S., Surarit, R., Soo-ampon, S and Kasetsuwan, R. 2000 Fluoride in water consumed by children in remote areas of Thailand. *Southeast Asian Journal of Tropical Medicine and Public Health,* **31**(2), 319–324.

Cortes, D.F., Ellwood, R.P., O'Mullane, D.M. and de Magalhaes Bastos, J.R. 1996 Drinking water fluoride levels, dental fluorosis and caries experience in Brazil. *Journal of Public Health Dentistry,* **56**(4), 226–228.

Dean, H.T. 1933 Distribution of mottled enamel in the United States. *Public Health Reports,* **48**(25), 703–734.

Dean, H.T. 1938 Endemic fluorosis and its relation to dental caries. *Public Health Reports,* **53**, 1443–1452.

Dean, H.T. 1945 On the epidemiology of fluorine and dental caries. In: Gies W.J. (Ed) *Fluorine in Dental Public Health*. New York Institute of Clinical Oral Pathology, New York, 19–30.

Dean, H.T. and Dixon, R.M. 1935 Mottled enamel in Texas. *Public Health Reports,* **50**(13), 424–442.

Dean, H.T. and Elvove, E. 1939 Mottled enamel in South Dakota. *Public Health Reports,* **54**, 212–228.

Díaz-Barriga, F., Navarro-Quezada, A., Grijalva, M.I., Grimaldo, M., Loyola-Rodriguez, J.P. and Ortz, M.D. 1997a Endemic fluorosis in Mexico. *Fluoride,* **30**(4), 233–239.

Díaz-Barriga, F., Leyva, R., Quistían, J., Loyola-Rodríguez, J.P., Pozos, A. and Grimaldo, M. 1997b Endemic fluorosis in San Luis Potosi, Mexico. IV Source of fluoride exposure. *Fluoride,* **30**(4), 219–222.

Dissanayake, C.B. 1996 Water quality and dental health in the Dry Zone of Sri Lanka. *Environmental Geochemistry and Health, Geological Society Special Publication,* **113**, 131–140.

Driscoll, W.S., Horowitz, H.S., Meyers, R.J., Heifetz, S.B., Kingman, A. and Zimmerman, E.R. 1983 Prevalence of dental caries and dental fluorosis in areas with optimal and above-optimal water fluoride concentrations. *Journal of the American Dental Association,* **107**, 42–47.

Droste, R.L. 1987 *Fluoridation in Canada as of December 31, 1986.* Health and Welfare Canada, Ottawa, Ontario (IWE-AR WQB-89-154).

Fendall, N.R.E. and Grounds, J.G. 1965 The incidence and epidemiology of disease in Kenya, Part 1. Some diseases of social significance. *Journal of Tropical Medicine and Hygiene,* **68**, 77–84.

Fluoride Action Network 2001 *Fluoride pollution causes bone disease.* (http://www.fluoridealert.org/news/pakistan/lahore.htm).

FRRDF 1999 *State of Art Report on the Extent of Fluoride in Drinking Water and the Resulting Endemicity in India.* Fluorosis Research and Rural Development Foundation, New Delhi.

Grafe, E.M. and Dominok, G.W. 1978 [Bone fluorosis]. *Zeitschrift fur die gesamte innere Medizin und ihre Grenzgebiete,* **33**, 866–869. [In German].

Grech, P. 1966 Fluorosis in young persons – A further survey in northern Tanganyika, Tanzania. *British Journal of Radiology,* **39**, 761–764.

Grimaldo, M., Borja-Aburto, V.H., Ramírez, A.L., Ponce, M., Rosas, M and Díaz-Barriga, F. 1995 Endemic fluorosis in San Luis Potosi, Mexico. *Environmental Research,* **68**, 25–30.

Grobler, S.R., Dreyer, A.G. and Blignaut, R.J. 2001 Drinking water in South Africa: implications for fluoride supplementation. *Journal of the South African Dental Association,* **56**(11), 557–559.

Grobler, S.R., Louw, A.J. and van Kotze, T.J. 2001 Dental fluorosis and caries experience in relation to three different drinking water fluoride levels in South Africa. *International Journal of Paediatric Dentistry,* **11**(5), 372–379.

Gupta, S.C. 1999 Occurrence and management of high fluoride ground waters in Rajasthan. In: Proceedings of the National Seminar Fluoride Contamination, Fluorosis and Defluoridation Techniques, Udaipur, 6–9.

Haimanot, R.T., Fekadu, A. and Bushra, B. 1987 Endemic fluorosis in the Ethiopian Rift Valley. *Tropical and Geographical Medicine,* **39**(3): 209–217.

Hardisson, A., Rodriguez, M.I., Burgos, A., Flores, L.D., Gutierrez, R. and Varela, H. 2001 Fluoride levels in publically supplied and bottled drinking waters in the island of Tenerife, Spain. *Bulletin of Environmental Contamination and Toxicology,* **67**(2), 163–170.

Health Canada 1993 *Inorganic Fluorides*. Canadian Environmental Protection Act. Priority Substances List Assessment Report. Minister or Supply and Services Canada 1993, Ottawa, Canada.

Heikens, A., Sumarti, S., van Bergen, M., Widianarko, B., Fokkert, L., van Leeuwen, K. and Seinen, W. 2005 The impact of the hyperacid Ijen Crater Lake: risks of excess fluoride to human health. *Science of the Total Environment,* **346**, 56–69.

Hurtado, R. and Gardea-Torresdey, J. 2004 Environmental evaluation of fluoride in drinking water at "Los Altos de Jalisco", in the central Mexico region. *Journal of Toxicology and Environmental Health, Part A,* **67**, 1741–1753.

Ishii, T. and Suckling, G. 1991 The severity of dental fluorosis in children exposed to water with a high fluoride content for various periods of time. *Journal of Dental Research,* **70**(6), 952–956.

Ismail, A.I. and Messer, J.G. 1996 The risk of fluorosis in students exposed to a higher than optimal concentration of fluoride in well water. *Journal of Public Health Dentistry,* **56**(1), 22–27.

Jin, C., Yan, Z., Jianwei, L., Ruodeng, X. and Sangbu, D. 2000 Environmental fluoride content in Tibet. *Environmental Research,* **83**(3), 333–337.

Kaseva, M.E. 1993 Human exposure to excessive fluorides through 'Magadi' in Arumeru Area, Northern Tanzania. Proceedings of the Joint TPHA 12th Annual and ECSAPHA 2nd Biennial Scientific Conference, October 25–29, Arusha International Conference Centre, Arusha, Tanzania.

Kodali, V.R.R., Krishnamachari, K.A.V.R. and Gowrinathsastry, J. 1994 Detrimental effects of high fluoride concentrations in drinking water on teeth in an endemic fluorosis area in South India. *Tropical Doctor,* **24**, 136–137.

Lester, F.T. 1974 Fluorotic myelopathy – A rare case, with a review of the literature. *Ethiopian Medical Journal,* **12**, 39–49.

Liang, C. 1998 [Evaluation on the effects of water defluoridation measures in China.] *Wei Sheng Yan Jiu,* **27**(1), 16–28. Article in Chinese.

Liang, C., Ji, R. and Cao, S. 1997 Epidemiological analysis of endemic fluorosis in China. *Environmental Carcinogenicity and Ecotoxicological Reviews,* **C15**(2), 123–138.

Malde, M.K., Zerihun, L., Julshamn, J. and Bjorvatn, K. 2004 Fluoride, calcium and magnesium intake in children living in a high-fluoride area in Ethiopia. Intake through food. *International Journal of Paediatric Dentistry,* **14**, 167–174.

Manji, F., Baelum, V. and Fejerskov, O. 1986a Dental fluorosis in an area of Kenya with 2 ppm fluoride in the drinking water. *Journal of Dental Research,* **65**(5), 659–62.

Manji, F., Baelum, V., Fejerskov, O. and Gemert, W. 1986b Enamel changes in two low-fluoride areas of Kenya. *Caries Research,* **20**, 371–380.

Manji, F., Baelum, V. and Fejerskov, O. 1986c Fluoride, altitude and dental fluorosis. *Caries Research,* **20**, 473–480.

Mauguhan-Brown, H. 1935 Our Land. Is our population satisfactory? The results of inspection of school ages. *South African Medical Journal,* **9**, 822.

McCaffrey, L.P. 1995 Distribution and origin of high fluoride groundwater in the Western Bushveld Areas. In: *Fluoride and Fluorosis: The Status of South African Research 1995,* 2.

McCaffrey, L.P. and Willis, J.P. 1997 Distribution and origin of fluoride in rural drinking water supplies in the Western Bushveld Areas of South Africa. In: *4th International Symposium on Environmental Geochemistry 1997,* 62.

Meenakshi, V.K., Garg, Kavita, Renuka and Anju Malik 2004 Groundwater quality in some villages of Haryana, India: focus on fluoride and fluorosis. *Journal of Hazardous Materials,* **106B**, 85–97.

Milgalter, N., Zadik, D. and Kelman, A.M. 1974 Fluorosis and dental caries in Yotvata area. *Israel Dental Journal,* **23**, 104–109.

Ministry of Water Resources 2004 Contamination of water sources. Press Release of the Government of India, Ministry of Water Resources, Rajya Sabha, *Hindustan Times*, 8 December 2004

Mjengera, H.J. 1988 Excess fluoride in potable water and defluoridation technology, with emphasis on the use of polyaluminium, chloride and magnetite. Tampere University of Technology.

MMWR 1999 Fluoridation of drinking water to prevent dental caries. *Morbidity and Mortality Weekly Report,* **48** (41), 933–940.

Moola, M.H. 1996 Fluoridation in South Africa. *Community Dental Health*, **13**(Suppl. 2), 51–55.

Mosha, H.J. 1984 Endemic dental fluorosis and the possibilities of defluoridation and fluoridation of water supplies in Tanzania. *Odonto-Stomatologie Tropicale,* **7**(2), 89–96.

Nair, K.R. and Manji, F. 1982 Endemic fluorosis in deciduous dentition – A study of 1276 children in typically high fluoride area (Kiambu) in Kenya. *Odonto-Stomatologie Tropicale,* **4**, 177–184.

Nair, K.R., Manji, F. and Gitonga, J.N. 1984 The occurrence and distribution of fluoride in groundwaters in Kenya. In: *Challenges in African Hydrology and Water Resources* (Proceedings of the Harare Symposium). IAHS Publications 144, 75–86.

Ncube, E.J. and Schutte, C.F. 2005 The occurrence of fluoride in South African groundwater: A water quality and health problem. *Water SA* **31**(1), 35–40.

Nevill, L.B. and Brass, W. 1953 Preliminary report on dental fluorosis in Kenyan European children. *East African Medical Journal,* **30**(6), 235–242.

Noppakun, W., Ratanasthein, B., Prapamontol, T., Asanchinda, P., Obsuwan, K., Na Suwan, J. and Promputha, M. 2000 Impact assessement of geothermal source to fluorosis in Doi Hang subdistrict, Muang district, Chiangrai Province. In: *Proceedings of the third international workshop on fluorosis and defluoridation of water.* Chaingmai, Thailand, November 20–24, 2000.

Ockerse, T. 1944 Incidence of dental caries among school children in South Africa. Government Printer, Pretoria.

Ockerse, T. 1949 Dental Caries chemical and experimental investigations. Thesis submitted for D.Sc. University of Pretoria, South Africa.

Olsson, B. 1978 Dental findings in high-fluoride areas in Ethiopia. *Community Dentistry and Oral Epidemiology,* **7**, 51–56.

Ortiz, D., Castro, L., Turrubiartes, F., Milam, J. and Díaz-Barriga, F. 1998 Assessment of the exposure to fluoride from drinking water in Durango, Mexico, using a geographical information system. *Fluoride,* **31**(4), 183–187.

Paoloni, J.D., Fiorentino, C.E., Sequeira, M.E. 2003 Fluoride contamination of aquifers in the southeast subhumid pampa, Argentina. *Environmental Toxicology*, **18**(5), 317–320.

Prasertsom, P. 1998 Fluoride used for caries prevention. *Fact Sheet – Dental Health,* **1**(4), 1–4.

Public Health Service 1962 *Public Health Service drinking water standards – revised 1962.* Washington, DC. US Department of Health, Education and Welfare. PHS publication no. 956.

Queste, A., Lacombe, M., Hellmeier, W., Hillermann, F., Bortulussi, B., Kaup, M., Ott, K. and Mathys, W. 2001 High concentrations of fluoride and boron in drinking water wells in the Muenster region – results of a preliminary investigation. *International Journal of Environmental Health,* **203**(3), 221–224.

Reddy, N.B. and Prasad, K.S.S. 2003 Pyroclastic fluoride in ground waters in some parts of Tadpatri Taluk, Anantapur district, Andhra Pradesh. *Indian Journal of Environmental Health,* **45**(4), 285–288.

Reimann, C., Bjorvatn, K., Frengstad, B., Melaku, Z., Tekle-Haimanot, R. and Siewers, U. 2003 Drinking water quality in the Ethiopian section of the East African Rift valley I – data and health aspects. *Science of the Total Environment,* **311**, 65–80.

Rwenyonyi, C M; Birkeland, J M; Haugejorden, O; Bjorvatn, K 2000 Age as a determinant of severity of dental fluorosis in children residing in areas with 0.5 and 2.5 mg fluoride per liter in drinking water. *Clinical Oral Investigations,* **4**(3), 157–161.

Rwenyonyi, C., Bjorvatn, K., Birkeland, J. and Haugejorden, O. 1998 Altitude as a risk indicator of dental fluorosis in children residing in areas with 0.5 and 2.5 mg fluoride per litre in drinking water. *Caries Research,* **33**(4), 267–274.

Saparamadu, D.G. 2000 An overview of the de-fluoridation project in Sri Lanka – some experiences. In: *Proceedings of the third international workshop on fluorosis and defluoridation of water.* Chaingmai, Thailand, November 20–24, 2000.

Segreto, V.A., Collins, E.M., Camann, D and Smith, C.T. 1984 A current study of mottled enamel in Texas. *Journal of the American Dental Association,* **108**, 56–59.

Shah, M.T. and Danishwar, S. 2003 Potential fluoride contamination in the drinking water of Naranji area, Northwest Frontier Province, Pakistan. *Environmental Geochemistry and Health,* **25**, 475–481.

Short, H.E., Pandit, C.G. and Taghavachari, T.N. 1937 Endemic fluorosis in Nellore District of South India. *Indian Medical Gazette,* **72**, 396–398.

Smith, D.A., Harris, H.A. and Kirk, R. 1953 Fluorosis in the Butana, Sudan. *Journal of Tropical Medicine and Hygiene,* **56**, 57–58.

Srikanth, R., Viswanatham, K.S., Kahsai, F., Fisahatsion, A and Asmellash, M. 2002 Fluoride in groundwater in selected villages in Eritrea (North East Africa). *Environmental Monitoring and Assessment,* **75**(2), 169–177.

Staz, J. 1938 Dental caries in South Africa. *South African Journal of Medical Science,* **3**, 2–25.

Toshikazu, W., Takashi, K., Shinji, A, Mitsuru, A., Kenji, T., Shiro, S., Ji, R and Liange, C. 2000 Skeletal fluorosis from indoor burning of coal in southwestern China. *Fluoride,* **33**(3), 135–139.

Tsutsui, A., Yagi, M and Horowitz, A.M. 2000 The prevalence of dental caries and fluorosis in Japanese communities with up to 1.4 ppm of naturally occurring fluoride. *Journal of Public Health Dentistry,* **60**(3), 147–153.

Vaish, A.K. and Vaish, P. 2000 Fluoride contamination, fluorosis and defluoridation at domestic level: a case study from Dungarpur district, Rajasthan, India. In: Proceedings of the third international workshop on fluorosis and defluoridation of water. Chiangmai, Thailand, November 20–24, 2000.

Wang, C.S., Bu, X.H. and Gu, T.D. 1997 The epidemiological study of endemic fluorosis in Huai-bei region, Jiangsu province. *Zhing Guo Di Fang Bing Xue Zha Zhi Supplement,* **12**(4-A), 10–13.

Wang, L.F. and Huang, J.Z. 1995 Outline of control practice of endemic fluorosis in China. *Social Science and Medicine,* **41**(8), 1191–1195.

WHO 1996 *Guidelines for Drinking-Water Quality. Second Edition. Volume 2, Health criteria and other supporting information.* World Health Organization, Geneva.

WHO 2004 *Guidelines for Drinking-Water Quality. Volume 1 Recommendations.* 3rd edition, World Health Organization, Geneva.

Williamson, M.M. 1953 Endemic dental fluorosis in Kenya a preliminary report. *The East African Medical Journal,* **30**(6), 217–233.

Wondwossen, F., Åstrøm, A.N., Bjorvatn, K. and Bårdsen, A. 2004 The relationship between dental caries and dental fluorosis in areas with moderate- and high-fluoride drinking water in Ethiopia. *Community Dentistry and Oral Epidemiology,* **32**, 337–344.

Wongdem, J.G., Aderinokun, G.A., Sridhar, M.K. and Selkur, S. 2000 Prevalence and distribution pattern of enamel fluorosis in Langtang town, Nigeria. *African Journal of Medicine and Medical Science,* **29**, 243–246.

Yadav, J.P. and Lata, S. 2003 Urinary fluoride levels and prevalence of dental fluorosis in children of Jhajjar District, Haryana. *Indian Journal of Medical Science,* **57**(9), 394–399.

Yadav, S., Khan, T.I., Gupta, S., Gupta, A.B. and Yadava, R.N. 1999 Fluorosis in India with special reference to Rajasthan. In: Proceedings of the International Conference on Water, Environment, Ecology, Socioeconomics and Health Engineering (WEESHE), Seoul National University, 18–21st October, 3–10.

Zhang, B., Hong, M., Zhao, Y., Lin, X., Zhang, X. and Dong, J. 2003 Distribution and risk assessment of fluoride in drinking water in the West Plain region of Jilin Province, China. *Environmental Geochemistry and Health* **25**, 421–431.

Zheng, B. and Hong, Y. 1988 Chapter 9 Geochemical environment related to human endemic fluorosis in China. In: *Geochemistry and Health,* Edited by Thornton, I. with assistance from Doyle, H. and Moir, A. Northwood, 93–96.

Ziegler, J. 2002 United Nations Economic and Social Council. Report E/CN.4/2002/58/Add.1.

Appendix

Indices of severity of dental fluorosis

The following are some examples of the more commonly used indices of dental fluorosis.

Dean's Index

After Dean *et al*. (1935)

1. Normal
2. Questionable
   A few white flecks to occasional white spots.
3. Very Mild
   Less than 25 per cent of the tooth surfaces covered by small white opaque areas.
4. Mild
   Fifty per cent of the tooth surfaces covered by white opaque areas.

5. Moderate
Nearly all the tooth surfaces are involved, with minute pitting and brown or yellowish stains.
6. Severe
Smoky white appearance of all the teeth with hypoplasia, chipping and large brown stains, which vary from chocolate brown to black. There is discreet and confluent pitting, often accompanied by attrition.

DDE (Developmental Defects of Enamel) Index

After Fédération Dentaire Internationale (1992)

A simplified version of this Index categorizes three broad types of defect: diffuse opacities, demarcated opacities and hypoplasias.

Terminology used to describe enamel defects
After Holloway and Ellwood (1997)
1. Diffuse opacity
Opacity with poorly defined boundary, which merges into the surrounding enamel.
2. Demarcated opacity
Opacity with clearly defined boundary from adjacent enamel.
3. Hypomineralized enamel
Incompletely mineralized enamel.
4. Developmental defects of enamel
Disturbance in hard tissue matrices and their mineralization during odontogenesis.
5. Hypoplasia
Quantitative defect in enamel, reduced thickness of enamel.
6. Opacity
Qualitative defect in enamel, abnormality in translucency of enamel.

Thylstrup and Fejerskov (TF) Index

After Thylstrup and Fejerskov (1978)

Score 0
Normal translucency of enamel remains after prolonged air-drying.
Score 1
Narrow white lines located corresponding to the perikymata.

Score 2
Smooth surfaces

More pronounced lines of opacity which follow the perikymata. Occasional confluence of adjacent lines.

Occlusal surfaces

Scattered areas of opacity <2 mm in diameter and pronounced opacity of cuspal ridges.

Score 3
Smooth surfaces

Merging and irregular cloudy areas of opacity. Accentuated drawing of perikymata often visible between opacities.

Occlusal surfaces

Confluent areas of marked opacity. Worn areas appear almost normal but usually circumscribed by a rim of opaque enamel.

Score 4
Smooth surfaces

The entire surface exhibits marked opacity or appears chalky white. Parts of surface exposed to attrition appear less affected.

Occlusal surface

Entire surface exhibits marked opacity. Attrition is often pronounced shortly after eruption.

Score 5
Smooth and occlusal surfaces

Entire surface displays marked opacity with focal loss of outermost enamel (pits) <2 mm in diameter.

Score 6
Smooth surfaces

Pits are regularly arranged in horizontal bands <2 mm in vertical extension.

Occlusal surfaces

Confluent areas <3 mm in diameter exhibit loss of enamel. Marked attrition.

Score 7
Smooth surfaces

Loss of outermost enamel in irregular areas involving <½ of entire surface.

Occlusal surfaces

Changes in the morphology caused by merging pits and marked attrition.

Score 8
Smooth and occlusal surfaces

Loss of outermost enamel involving >½ of surface

Score 9
Smooth and occlusal surfaces

Loss of main part of enamel with change in anatomic appearance of surface. Cervical rim of almost unaffected enamel is often noted.

TSIF (Tooth Surface Index of Fluorosis)

After Horowitz *et al*. (1984)

Score 0
Enamel shows no evidence of fluorosis.

Score 1
Enamel shows definite evidence of fluorosis, namely areas with parchment-white colour that total less than one-third of the visible enamel surface. This category includes fluorosis confined only to incisal edges of anterior teeth and cusp tips of posterior teeth ("snowcapping").

Score 2
Parchment-white fluorosis totals at least one-thirds of the visible surface, but less than two-thirds.

Score 3
Parchment-white fluorosis totals at least two-thirds of the visible surface.

Score 4
Enamel shows staining in conjunction with any of the preceding levels of fluorosis. Staining is defined as an area of definite discolouration that may range from light to very dark brown.

Score 5
Discrete pitting of the enamel exists, unaccompanied by evidence of staining of intact enamels. A pit is defined as a definite physical defect in the enamel surface with a rough floor that is surrounded by a wall of intact enamel. The pitted area is usually stained or differs in colour from the surrounding enamel.

Score 6
Both discrete pitting and staining of the intact enamel exist.

Score 7
Confluent pitting of the enamel surface exists. Large areas of enamel may be missing and the anatomy of the tooth may be altered. Dark-brown stain is usually present.

References

Dean, H.T., Dixon, R.M. and Cohen, C. 1935 Mottled enamel in Texas. *Public Health Reports*, **50**(13), 424–442.

Fédération Dentaire Internationale 1992 A review of the developmental defects of enamel index (DDE Index). Commission on Oral Health, Research and Epidemiology. *International Dental Journal*, **42**, 411–426.

Holloway, P.J. and Ellwood, R.P. 1997 The prevalence, cause and cosmetic importance of dental fluorosis in the United Kingdom: review. *Community Dental Health*, **14**, 148–155.

Thylstrup, A. and Fejerskov, O. 1978 Clinical appearance of dental fluorosis in permanent teeth in relation to histologic changes. *Community Dentistry and Oral Epidemiology,* **6**, 315–328.

Horowitz, H.S., Heifetz, S.B., Driscoll, W.S., Kingman, A. and Meyers, R.J. 1984 A new method for assessing the prevalence of dental fluorosis – the Tooth Surface Index of fluorosis. *Journal of the American Dental Association,* **109**, 37–41.

Index